BLACK AND PREGNANT IN AMERICA

Temitope Oluyemo

Dedication

This book is a heartfelt tribute to every extraordinary Black woman out there. To those who have encountered immense challenges yet continue to rise and fight, and to those who have tragically lost their lives in that very battle. I want each and every one of you to know that you are warriors, deserving of nothing but the absolute best.

In a world that sometimes seeks to diminish our worth, we rise above. We are not just ordinary beings; we possess a strength that transcends the boundaries of what is considered human. We are superhumans, capable of bringing forth life into this world, nurturing it with love, and guiding it with wisdom.

Our journey has been marked by both triumphs and trials. We have faced adversity with unwavering resolve and have emerged stronger, wiser, and more resilient. We have shattered glass ceilings, dismantled barriers, and rewritten the narratives that once sought to confine us.

We carry within us the legacy of our ancestors, the indomitable spirit of those who came before us. We are the embodiment of their hopes, dreams, and aspirations. With every step we take, we honor their sacrifices and pave the way for generations yet to come.

But let us also acknowledge the rawness of our experiences. The pain, the sorrow, the burden we often carry on our shoulders. We have been overlooked, underestimated, and silenced for far too long. We have been the victims of systemic injustice and racial prejudice.

Yet, despite it all, we rise. We rise with a fiery determination, fueled by the knowledge that we are deserving of respect, equality, and love. We rise to create a world where our daughters and granddaughters can walk freely, unencumbered by the chains of discrimination.

This book is a celebration of our greatness, a testament to the power and beauty that resides within each of us. It is a reminder that we are not alone in this journey. We stand united, hand in hand, supporting one another as we navigate the complexities of life.

To every Black woman reading these words, know that you are seen, you are valued, and you are loved. Your presence in this world is a gift, and your contributions have the power to change it for the better.

May this book serve as a beacon of hope, inspiration, and empowerment. May it ignite a fire within you, reminding you of your inherent strength and reminding the world of the greatness that lies within every Black woman.

We are warriors, and together, we will continue to rise.

Table Of Contents

Introduction

In the tapestry of American society, where dreams and aspirations are woven, a darker thread quietly unravels the experiences of a remarkable group of women. Amidst the euphoria and tender hopes accompanying pregnancy, a different hue emerges for black mothers-to-be in the United States.

Their journey is a symphony of resilience, grit, and an unjust disparity reverberating nationwide. These women embark on a poignant and captivating narrative in a land where equality and opportunity should reign supreme. This tale unveils the arduous path of being pregnant and black in America.

From the first flicker of life within, these courageous women navigate a labyrinth of challenges that surpass the ordinary trials of pregnancy. While embracing the profound joy of new beginnings, they bear the weight of historical injustices, systemic prejudices, and entrenched biases that penetrate the fabric of their daily existence. Celebrating new life intertwines with the stark reality of racial disparities in maternal healthcare, unequal access to quality prenatal care, and alarming pregnancy-related complications and mortality rates.

Yet, their spirits remain unyielding through it all, fortified by an unwavering resilience that inspires and tugs at the heartstrings.

They navigate a healthcare system that often overlooks their distinctive needs, where unconscious biases can dictate the level of care they receive.

They confront harmful stereotypes perpetuating fear, mistrust, and discrimination narratives. And yet, amidst these trials, they stand firm, drawing strength from the bonds of their community, the richness of their culture, and the boundless love they hold for their unborn children.

This is not just their story—a call to action that demands our unwavering attention. It beckons us to confront the inequities that mar our society, challenge the prevailing norms, and dismantle the systemic barriers that obstruct the safe and joyous pregnancy journey for black women in America. It is an invitation to embark on a shared voyage of empathy, education, and advocacy for transformative change.

Prepare to be captivated as we traverse this path together—expect to be enlightened, moved, and profoundly challenged. Brace yourself for a tapestry woven with raw emotions, unspoken truths, and an unyielding spirit that echoes through the voices of those who have witnessed the intersection of pregnancy and blackness in America.

Through their stories, we can reshape our collective understanding, ignite our compassion, and inspire tireless efforts toward a future where every expectant mother, irrespective of race, can embark on the pregnancy journey with hope, dignity, and unwavering support.

So, open your heart and mind, and let us embark on this compelling journey together. Let us illuminate the shadows, shatter the barriers, and ensure that the experience of being pregnant and black in America becomes a tale of adversity and a triumph of resilience, equity, and justice.

Hurray! You're pregnant. You can't wait to see that bundle of joy. You can't wait to have him in your arms and see that warm, innocent smile. Days keep rolling by as you can no longer hide the excitement of seeing your new baby. You've got baby clothes and all the other things you'll need for you and your baby.

You count each day till your delivery date in excitement as you begin to picture how you'll react when you first hold your newborn baby in your arms. Although you're feeling the contractions little by little, they tell you that your baby's sunshine can come anytime soon. You're about to experience the joy of motherhood.

You take short walks around the house when you feel the wetness drip down your thigh — it is time! You brace yourself for what's coming as you get rushed to the hospital.

But you get the shocker of your life; you're asked to wait even though they can see you're in pain. The doctors and nurses keep attending to other people while you lay on the hospital bed, every inch of your body jolting with pain.

They came to tell you that you were even lucky they attended to you, and you see preferential treatment comprehensive and transparent. And the worst feeling of all is you get racially profiled.

But what about you? And your baby? Your life? Your baby's life?

Doesn't it matter at all?

The mortality rate for most black women during pregnancy and childbirth in the United States is substantially higher when compared to white women. Research conducted by the Centers for Disease Control and Prevention (CDC) made known the maternal mortality rate for black women is approximately triple times higher than that of white women. I experienced this forehand, having my third child in the United States.

To put all pleasantries aside, I will tell you a little about myself – my name is Temitope Oluyemo. I am a real estate agent in Georgia and a successful entrepreneur. A mother of three wonderful boys with whom I have dedicated my heart to giving the best life.

With this book, I want to share my birth experience and compare each birth experience with another. I also want to educate every black American and woman in the same shoes as mine. This book is also an eye-opener for those women who have yet to have a baby. The book would also serve as a public awareness to all who read and are ready to embark on the nine months journey of pregnancy. The reason for doing this is to let you fully understand the vast difference between them — my three children and their places of birth.

You may be wondering, what is different in having three childbirths? Yes, it's a whole lot different than you think. Asides the usual changes associated with pregnancy in the body. Before going into my personal experience with pregnancy and childbirth, let's understand the few changes in the body during pregnancy.

Twelve weeks into pregnancy, the increment of the uterus causes the woman's abdomen to protrude slightly. This is actually to make enough room for your baby – you don't want to have a baby squeezed up in your flat tummy, do you?

And even if you already have a big belly, that doesn't guarantee enough space to hold up a baby. That is why an increase in the uterus size is vital for a healthy baby. The uterus continues to enlarge throughout pregnancy. The now-growing uterus extends further to the lower level of the navel by 20 weeks and to the lower edge of the rib cage by 36 weeks.

Carrying a baby affects virtually every hormone in the body, most times due to the effects of particular hormones produced by the placenta. A good example, for instance, is the placenta makes ready a hormone that stimulates the woman's thyroid gland to become more effective than usual when she isn't with a child.

This produces more significant amounts of thyroid hormones around the body. Another noticeable change in a pregnant woman's body is the joints and ligaments in the woman's pelvis loosen and become more flexible. Just like enlarging the uterus, this change helps make room and prepare the woman to deliver the baby. However, this changes the woman's posture, and she will have to do some little exercise while maintaining a good diet to be more mobile with carrying the baby.

All these are regular changes every woman experiences within and during pregnancy, even though it varies from body to body. Around 2016, an image of two women close to childbirth, posing with their bellies pressed together, was on the air, and it sparked a lot of comments. One had a smaller stomach that didn't appear pregnant, and the other was already protruding, as most pregnant women's bellies do. There isn't anyone at first glance who wouldn't doubt they were both pregnant and, not to say, about the same time, far away. The difference was about four weeks apart, which freaked out the internet.

Why is this so important? – You might ask. These two women were both pregnant and not so far away from giving birth, yet they looked so utterly nothing alike I'm terms of belly size. Is one woman having a better dietician than the other? Or is the other just spending a lot of time at the gym? These questions are typical to pop up when addressing their case, but it has nothing to do with that.

This is just a natural but rare situation in pregnancy known as cryptic pregnancy, which the more petite belly woman has. In rarer cases, some people do not realize they are pregnant until about seven months into it. This can be surprising, but that's how it is. The human body varies from one to another, with one having a more muscular immune system and the other slightly weaker. Experimenting wouldn't be a bad idea; take two bottles of water and have a friend compete with you to finish your water bottles. This experiment aims to show how much water you can take in compared to how much another person can drink. Your drinking partner might be more minor or even more significant than you – that doesn't matter in winning the bout.

You might be surprised that the smaller one among you two could accommodate more water than the other. The best part is yet to come; look down at the sizes of your bellies and compare. One of you is sure to have a bigger tummy than the other – this mystery explains why it's like that with pregnant women. Just that it isn't a mystery. There are certain stages of pregnancy; that is how you know you are with a child.

Stages Of Pregnancy

Pregnancy lasts about 40 weeks, counting from the first day you survive your expected period. These weeks are divided into three trimesters. You discover what's happening with you and your baby during these trimesters. All women carry different baby bellies that can look like opposites, even at similar stages of pregnancy— and that's natural and healthy.

The expected first sign of pregnancy is missing a menstrual period or two or more in consecutive periods. When you haven't seen your period for the second or third time, it's only standard for you to see a doctor.

However, some women visit the hospital after missing one month of their menstrual flow. It is also important to note that many women experience other pregnancy symptoms before they miss a period. Missing a period does not always mean a woman is pregnant.

Menstrual fluctuations are common and can have several causes, including taking birth control pills, conditions such as polycystic ovary syndrome, bad food hygiene, and specific medications that might alter their hormonal functions. Women who miss a period should see their health advisor or doctor to find out whether they are pregnant or, possibly, if they have another health problem.

The early stages of pregnancy symptoms vary from woman to woman. A woman may experience every common symptom, just a few or none. Some signs of early pregnancy include the primary character of pregnancy missing a menstrual period or two or more consecutive periods. Still, many women experience other pregnancy symptoms before they miss a period. Some signs of early pregnancy include:

1. Slight bleeding

During pregnancy, approximately 25% of women may experience a phenomenon known as slight bleeding or spotting. This occurrence is characterized by lighter-colored blood compared to regular menstrual blood.

It commonly takes place around 6 to 12 days after conception, coinciding with the implantation of the fertilized egg. However, it's important to note that this type of bleeding can persist throughout the first 12 weeks of pregnancy.

This phenomenon holds educational and compelling value as it sheds light on a relatively common aspect of early pregnancy. By understanding that slight bleeding or spotting is possible, individuals can be better informed and prepared for the changes their bodies may undergo during this crucial period. Moreover, this knowledge empowers expectant mothers to differentiate between normal bleeding and potential complications, allowing them to seek appropriate medical advice when necessary.

2. Tender, Swollen Breasts Or Nipples.

Ladies, brace yourselves for some early signs of a life-changing journey! Around 1 to 2 weeks after conception, you might start noticing fascinating changes in your body. Get ready for an adventure as those hormones kick in and turn your world upside down, starting with your lovely bosom! Picture this: your breasts become the center of attention, tender and tingly, as if sending you secret messages of the miracle growing within.

They'll even feel a little fuller and heavier, giving you that delightful sensation of a beautiful transformation underway. Embrace this exciting phase, and it's time to treat yourself to a fresh collection of foam bras, ready to support your journey like never before!

3. Fatigue

Women may feel tired during early pregnancy because their bodies make more of a hormone called progesterone, which helps support the pregnancy and promotes the growth of milk glands in the breasts. Also, the body sends more blood to provide nutrients to the growing baby. Fatigue can be noticed by pregnant women as early as one week after coconception.

4. Headaches

During early pregnancy, the sudden rise of hormones, particularly estrogen, and progesterone, can contribute to headaches in some women. While pregnancy headaches are generally considered normal, it is essential to monitor their severity and frequency and consult a healthcare provider if there are any concerns.

5. Nausea and vomiting

Did you know pregnancy can bring on a not-so-fun surprise known as "morning sickness"? But here's the twist: it can strike any time of the day! This symptom can start two weeks after conception and stick around throughout pregnancy.

Now, picture going through all that and then being treated differently just because of your skin color. It's a bummer. Well, sadly, that's the reality for many Black women. They face a higher risk of pregnancy-related complications and even mortality compared to White women. But why does this happen? Let's dig into it!

The issue of maternal mortality is complex, but one major factor is something called systemic racism and discrimination. It's like an invisible monster that affects the health outcomes of Black women.

For instance, Black women are less likely to receive the proper prenatal care they need. They are more prone to health problems like high blood pressure, gestational diabetes, and pre-eclampsia during pregnancy.

But it doesn't stop there. Black women are more likely to face economic challenges and have limited access to quality healthcare. And guess what? That increases their risk for pregnancy-related complications even more. It's not fair, but it's the unfortunate truth.

To make matters worse, evidence suggests that some healthcare providers unknowingly hold biases and treat Black women differently. It's called implicit bias, which can lead to suboptimal care. It's like having a hidden obstacle course during pregnancy.

But fear not! We can turn this around. The high maternal mortality rate for Black women is a health problem and a matter of justice. It's time to take action and tackle this issue head-on.

So, what can we do? We need a comprehensive approach! Let's fight systemic racism and discrimination, ensuring women have equal access to quality healthcare. Let's invest in programs and policies that support the health and well-being of Black women and their families. By addressing these underlying factors, we can ensure every woman has a safe and healthy pregnancy journey.

See learning about these things doesn't have to be a drag. It's all about understanding the challenges and working together to improve things. Together, we can create a future where all women have a fair shot at a joyful and healthy pregnancy experience.

Chapter One

A Personal Journey Through Racism in Black Women's Pregnancy

In 2011, I welcomed my first child into the world in a general hospital in Nigeria. Four years later, in 2015, I gave birth to my second child at Grady Hospital in Atlanta, Georgia. Then, in 2022, my journey took an unexpected turn when I discovered I was pregnant again while experiencing what I thought was a stomach ulcer.

On a seemingly ordinary day in March, feeling unwell and relying on over-the-counter medications like Zantac and Omeprazole for my assumed ulcer, a friend suggested that I take a pregnancy test. Despite being confident that pregnancy was unlikely, I decided to try it to rule it out. To my utter surprise, the examination revealed that I was indeed pregnant.

The news took me aback. Pregnancy was not part of my plans as I had been dieting and exercising, preparing for my upcoming 40th birthday.

Nonetheless, I embraced the joy that came with the unexpected news. Excited about the journey ahead, I started looking for insurance and sought a doctor's office attached to a nearby hospital to ensure the best care for myself and my baby.

A routine urine test was conducted during my first visit to the clinic. The doctor informed me that they had detected protein in my urine and suggested it could indicate either kidney stones or preeclampsia.

Further tests were necessary to determine the underlying cause. Confusion washed over me as I worried about the well-being of my unborn child. Reluctantly, I signed documents accepting the additional tests, even though my insurance didn't cover them.

And so, the series of medical investigations began. From multiple visits to the lab for tests to frequent blood samples, I soon found myself experiencing the consequences of excessive blood work. As a result, I became anemic during the early stages of pregnancy.

This meant my baby wasn't receiving sufficient iron, B12, and folic acid crucial for healthy development. Despite my struggles to eat due to common pregnancy symptoms like morning sickness, I knew my body could sustain a pregnancy, as I had done it twice before.

Curiously, I was asked to undergo a 24-hour urine test to evaluate my kidneys, which yielded average results. The doctor then prescribed baby aspirin as a preventive measure against preeclampsia.

Additionally, he inquired about my exposure to chickenpox and even suggested that I might be a carrier of sickle cell anemia. To confirm this, they insisted on testing the baby's father, adding further financial burden.

At that moment, it became clear to me that something was amiss. How could a well-educated, 39-year-old woman with a Bachelor's degree be unaware of being a sickle cell carrier? Did being of African descent automatically imply having sickle cell anemia? The situation felt unfair and unjust. I couldn't bear the thought of risking my life or my baby's life due to assumptions and biases based on my race.

Frustrated and concerned, I decided I would never return to that medical facility. The potential consequences of their actions on my unborn child were too significant a risk to take. It highlighted a systemic issue in the American healthcare system where black women are undervalued and their concerns often dismissed.

Considering my options, I contemplated returning to Grady Hospital, despite the hour-long drive from my new neighborhood. However, I resolved to wait until I reached 20 weeks of pregnancy before seeking their care.

In the meantime, I didn't take the aspirin because my blood pressure was normal, measuring 125/70, which is considered healthy for a pregnant woman. When I switched to a new doctor, I was shocked to learn that the aspirin I had been advised to take was harmful to my pregnancy.

Unlike my previous pregnancies, where I experienced no severe complications, this time, I found myself anemic due to the excessive blood work I had undergone within a short period. To make matters worse, I accumulated a staggering medical bill of $4000 in just a month, even after accounting for my insurance coverage.

It was disheartening to realize that in today's world, with all the advancements and progress, black women are still subjected to unfair treatment. It felt as though my life and the pain I was experiencing were being disregarded and dismissed.

The doctors seemed overly cautious, ordering countless tests and treatments for issues that didn't even exist. It felt like I was being treated like a mere lab specimen rather than a woman with previous pregnancy experiences and two healthy boys to care for. The thought of losing my life and leaving my children behind was unimaginable and terrifying.

Unfortunately, many black women don't have access to better healthcare for themselves and their babies. And even when they seek it out, they are often met with poor treatment and discrimination.

At 14 weeks, I underwent another round of tests to check for potential congenital disabilities and determine the baby's sex. To my surprise, I was required to register with a third-party lab that would charge me out-of-pocket for the tests.

This added to my fear and anxiety, as I worried about the potential complications these tests could pose to my baby. Endless questions filled my mind, and I sought solace in my children's presence, holding them tightly and frequently.

My thoughts grew darker, contemplating the possibility of my demise due to the complications I was being told I had. Was it preeclampsia? Kidney stones? Was my baby in danger due to my anemia? I even started considering writing a will, ensuring that my estate would be entrusted to my elder brother, an economist skilled in managing finances.

I knew my property would be safe with him. As for my children, I debated between leaving them in the care of my sister-in-law, my brother's wife, who I believed could care for them, or entrusting them to my Irish sister. Though I wasn't sure if my kids would want to move to Ireland, I couldn't help but plan for their future if I was no longer there to protect them.

I understand that reading these thoughts may seem peculiar, but I was genuinely terrified. I began organizing contingency plans to ensure my children would be cared for, even if I was no longer around. They were the reason I kept fighting and living each day.

When the doctors informed me about the need for another test at 20 weeks to screen for Down syndrome, I became skeptical. The previous test results indicated that everything was fine with the baby, yet they suggested injecting my belly and extracting fluids around it for further testing.

That was the moment I finally understood the message God had been trying to convey: I needed to run. I couldn't continue subjecting myself to costly tests that I had to pay for out-of-pocket.

Despite starting my pregnancy in good health, I feel incredibly unwell, as if I have fallen ill or contracted some unknown ailment. The concern for my baby's well-being overwhelms me, and I am determined to ensure that nothing jeopardizes their safety. Every symptom or discomfort I experience brings forth a wave of anxiety as I desperately seek reassurance that everything is alright within my growing belly.

This unexpected shift in my physical well-being has left me feeling bewildered and apprehensive. Each day presents new challenges, and I am acutely aware of the delicate balance between my health and the precious life inside me. The normalcy I once enjoyed has been replaced with a constant state of vigilance and a heightened sense of responsibility.

The relentless worry consumes me as I contemplate the potential risks and complications that could affect my baby. Every twinge, ache, or moment of fatigue sends me spiraling into a sea of doubts and fears. I meticulously monitor every aspect of my well-being, from my diet and exercise routine to my sleep patterns and stress levels. I am willing to do whatever it takes to safeguard the life that depends on me.

The anticipation of doctor's appointments and prenatal check-ups is comforting and anxiety-inducing. I yearn for medical professionals to offer insight into the mysterious ailments I am experiencing, alleviate my concerns, and provide guidance. Their expertise is a beacon of hope in this uncertain journey, a source of knowledge and expertise I desperately seek.

I long for the day when I can regain my vitality and well-being, when this cloud of sickness will dissipate, allowing me to enjoy the pregnancy miracle fully. Until then, I am determined to remain resilient and dedicated to preserving the health and safety of my unborn child.

My commitment to their well-being is unwavering. I will navigate this challenging period with the utmost care and vigilance, anticipating the joyous moment when I hold my healthy baby in my arms.

I will continue my story, but I must address every area of this recurring event and how to tackle them. Most expectant mothers, regardless of color or race, generally can look forward to a relatively complication-free pregnancy and the birth of a healthy baby. However, there is a possibility that all women might encounter the risk of developing medical problems or complications. For Black women, the risk is higher.

<h1 style="text-align:center">Chapter Two</h1>

<h2 style="text-align:center">Common Misconceptions of Black Women Pregnancies</h2>

There are some of the most common pregnancy complications in Black women, and this list can help you to be aware of what they are and how to get help immediately.

Preeclampsia or eclampsia

This can occur during or shortly after pregnancy. Preeclampsia can be a potentially dangerous complication involving a sudden spike in blood pressure. This condition can cause severe and sometimes fatal problems for the mother and the baby if not adequately monitored and managed. Severe preeclampsia can progress to eclampsia, where extremely high blood pressure can lead to coma or seizures.

What are the warning signs?

- High blood pressure.

- Severe headache.

- It is swelling in the hands, feet, face, or legs.

- Vision problems.

- Less frequent urination or smaller amounts than usual.

- Dark urine.

High Blood Pressure

High blood pressure sometimes develops in pregnancies but should also be monitored. However, if you have any signs of high blood pressure before pregnancy, it increases your risk of preeclampsia and preterm birth.

What are the warning signs?

According to the American Heart Association, high blood pressure doesn't usually come with symptoms. Regular blood pressure checks with an at-home pressure monitor or your doctor's office can help you monitor your blood pressure and let you know if you have it.

Gestational Diabetes

This mainly occurs in women that do not have diabetes before they are pregnant. This condition affects insulin, which helps your body use glucose (sugar) for energy. High blood sugar that is not carefully monitored and controlled can cause complications for you and your baby, so it is essential to take preventive steps.

What are the warning signs?

Gestational diabetes does not have specific symptoms, but your doctor should likely test you for the condition between the 24th and 28th weeks of pregnancy.

Postpartum Haemorrhage (PPH)

This is excessive bleeding after childbirth which can result in life-threatening loss of blood. PPH usually occurs after delivery within 24 hours of giving birth but can happen 12 weeks after having a baby. This has been a major cause of death in Black women as little or no attention is paid to them.

What are the warning signs?

It is normal to lose blood after pregnancy, but PPH is a medical emergency. These are signs to look out for, and when you experience any one of them you should go straight to see your health consultant.

- Feeling faint

- Blurred vision

- Chills

- Heavy nonstop vaginal bleeding

- Dizziness or confusion

- Nausea

- Weakness

- Rapid heartbeat.

Preterm labor

This happens when contractions start after the 20th week and before the 37th week of pregnancy. Babies born prematurely are more likely to develop serious long-term health problems if not carefully cared for.

What are the warning signs?

- Pelvic pressure

- Abdominal cramps

- Changes in the quantity of vaginal discharge

- Contractions that may/may not be painful

- Persistent backache

- Water breaking.

What Can You Do to Help Avoid Pregnancy Complications?

If you are or are looking to become pregnant, be proactive about your health, and take these three steps:

Ask relatives about any pregnancy problems they experienced. Some pregnancy complications run in families, giving valuable clues to your own risk. Act to minimize your risks with appropriate self-care and consistent prenatal/maternal care. Don't forget that you need ongoing care after your baby is born.

Advocate for yourself and your baby. Discuss any health concerns with your prenatal care provider right away.

With my research, I can only explain things that may help avoid pregnancy complications. Still, it's important to note that specific medical advice should always be sought from healthcare professionals who can consider individual circumstances.

Additionally, it's essential to address healthcare disparities and the unique experiences of Black American women concerning pregnancy. Black women in the United States face higher pregnancy complications and maternal mortality rates than other racial and ethnic groups. While addressing systemic issues is crucial, here are some general steps that may help promote a healthier pregnancy for Black American women:

1. Seek regular prenatal care: Early and regular prenatal care is vital for monitoring the health of both the mother and the baby. Establishing a relationship with a healthcare provider who understands Black American women's unique challenges and concerns can ensure that potential complications are identified and addressed promptly.

2. Find a culturally competent healthcare provider: Look for healthcare professionals knowledgeable about the specific health concerns and disparities affecting Black American women. Culturally qualified providers are more likely to understand and address their patient's unique needs and experiences, improving the quality of care received.

3. Educate yourself about pregnancy risks: Familiarize yourself with the common complications that can arise during pregnancy, such as gestational diabetes, preeclampsia, preterm labor, and postpartum depression. Being aware of the signs and symptoms can help you seek medical attention promptly if necessary.

4. Adopt a healthy lifestyle: Maintain a balanced diet of fruits, vegetables, whole grains, and lean proteins. Engage in regular physical activity unless otherwise advised by your healthcare provider. Avoid smoking, alcohol consumption, and illicit drugs, as they can increase the risk of pregnancy complications.

5. Address pre-existing medical conditions: If you have pre-existing health conditions such as hypertension, diabetes, or obesity, work closely with your healthcare provider to manage them effectively before and during pregnancy. Proper management can help reduce the risk of complications.

6. Address mental health concerns: Pregnancy can be emotionally challenging, and mental health is essential to overall well-being. Seek support from healthcare providers, therapists, or support groups if you experience anxiety, depression, or other mental health issues during or after pregnancy.

7. Advocate for yourself: Participate actively in your healthcare journey. If you have concerns or questions, don't hesitate to voice them and seek clarification. You deserve to be heard and treated with respect throughout your pregnancy and delivery.

8. Access support networks: Engage with community organizations, support groups, or online communities that provide resources and a supportive environment for Black American women.

Sharing experiences and information with others who have faced similar challenges can be empowering and help navigate potential pregnancy complications.

Remember, these general suggestions may not encompass the full range of considerations specific to Black American women's experiences. It's essential to consult with healthcare professionals who can provide personalized care and address the unique factors impacting the health of Black American women during pregnancy.

I repeatedly use the word "black," and you might wonder why. The reason is simple: black women in America often face distinct challenges when accessing healthcare. I believe so since my personal experience of being subjected to racial discrimination in a white hospital and how it made me feel like an object of curiosity rather than a patient in need of care. This painful encounter highlights racism, and black women must be prepared to fight for equality.

Chapter Three

Implicit Bias and Stereotypes in Obstetric Care

I vividly remember the day I entered the hospital, seeking medical attention. Even before the doctors attended to me, I was handed a symbolic card labeled "racial discrimination." It was as if my blackness had already predetermined the quality of care I would receive. The doctors' initial glances, filled with curiosity and detached scrutiny, made me feel like a specimen under examination rather than a human being in pain.

This experience was a stark reminder that racism continues to permeate the healthcare system, often leaving black women marginalized and ignored. The unequal treatment based on race can have devastating consequences for our well-being. It erodes our trust in the medical profession and adds stress and vulnerability to a challenging situation.

Black women should be ready to fight for equality because we deserve the same level of respect, dignity, and quality of care as anyone else. Our lives matter, and our voices must be heard. We must advocate for ourselves, demand equal treatment, and hold institutions accountable for their biases and discriminatory practices.

We must challenge the status quo and work towards dismantling the systemic barriers perpetuating racial healthcare disparities. By sharing our stories, raising awareness, and supporting organizations fighting racial justice, we can contribute to a future where black women no longer have to navigate a separate, unequal healthcare system.

Together, we can strive for a society that recognizes our worth, values our lives, and provides equal access to healthcare for all, regardless of the color of our skin. This brings me to the next topic of interest for black American women and humanists. Racism is a pest on our lovely soul that must be uprooted or watered down. There are adverse effects caused by racism and how it affects our healthcare services:

Racism and its Effect on healthcare systems

Racism has profound and far-reaching effects on healthcare systems and the health outcomes of marginalized communities, particularly in the context of maternal and infant health. Here are some ways in which racism impacts healthcare and exacerbates disparities in these areas:

1. Access to Care: Racism can create barriers to accessing healthcare services. Discriminatory practices such as racial profiling, bias in triaging, and unequal treatment contribute to disparities in access to quality prenatal care for pregnant individuals and appropriate healthcare for infants. Structural racism, including residential segregation, can limit the availability of healthcare facilities in marginalized communities.

2. Quality of Care: Implicit biases by healthcare providers can affect the quality of care provided to racial and ethnic minority patients. Studies have shown that racial and ethnic minorities, including pregnant individuals, may receive lower-quality care, experience longer wait times, and have their pain and symptoms underestimated or dismissed. These disparities can result in poorer health outcomes for both mothers and infants.

3. Maternal Mortality: Black and Indigenous women experience significantly higher maternal mortality rates than white women. Racial bias in healthcare can contribute to delays in diagnosing and treating conditions that can lead to maternal complications. Disparities in access to timely and appropriate prenatal care and lack of culturally competent care are also factors contributing to this issue.

4. Infant Mortality: Similar to maternal mortality, racial disparities in infant mortality rates are well-documented. Black infants, for instance, have consistently higher infant mortality rates than white infants. The complex interplay of social determinants of health, including racism, contributes to this disparity. Factors such as preterm birth, low birth weight, and inadequate postnatal care are more prevalent among racial and ethnic minority populations.

5. Stress and Mental Health: Experiences of racism and discrimination contribute to chronic stress among marginalized individuals, including pregnant individuals and new parents. This chronic stress can have negative impacts on maternal and infant health. Stress-related conditions, such as preterm labor and low birth weight, are more common in communities facing systemic racism.

Addressing these issues requires comprehensive strategies that acknowledge and actively work to dismantle racism in healthcare. Some potential solutions include:

1. Increasing Diversity in the Healthcare Workforce: Encouraging and supporting racial and ethnic diversity among healthcare providers can help foster culturally competent care and reduce biases.

2. Cultural Competency Training: Healthcare professionals should receive ongoing education and training to raise awareness of racial bias and cultural competence to provide equitable patient care.

3. Community Engagement and Outreach: Engaging with marginalized communities and involving them in decision-making can help address healthcare disparities. Developing trust and building partnerships can improve access to care and ensure community-specific needs are met.

4. Health Policy Reforms: Policies should be implemented to address the social determinants of health and reduce racial disparities in healthcare. This includes expanding access to affordable healthcare, promoting Medicaid expansion, and addressing structural racism in housing, education, and employment. Structural racism will be discussed later on, as it plays a massive role in the lives of black women

5. Data Collection and Research: Collecting and analyzing comprehensive data on race, ethnicity, and health outcomes is crucial to understanding and addressing healthcare disparities. Research on identifying the root causes and effective interventions is necessary to inform evidence-based policies and practices.

By recognizing and addressing the impact of racism on healthcare and maternal and infant health, societies can take significant steps toward achieving health equity and improving outcomes for all individuals, regardless of their race or ethnicity. As we work hard enough to battle the aftermath of racism we have to take note of the structural racism and understand why it's needed.

Structural racism refers to a system in which various aspects of society, including public policies, institutional practices, and cultural representations, contribute to reinforcing and perpetuating racial inequity. It is a deeply ingrained and pervasive form of racism that operates at both overt and covert levels, often leading to unequal outcomes and opportunities for different racial groups.

One of the key elements of structural racism is the presence of discriminatory public policies. These policies may be explicit or implicit and can be found in education, housing, criminal justice, employment, and healthcare. For example, redlining, a discriminatory housing practice historically prevalent in the United States, systematically denied loans and access to desirable neighborhoods to people of color. This resulted in the concentration of poverty and limited opportunities for upward mobility among marginalized communities.

Institutional practices also play a significant role in perpetuating structural racism. These practices are embedded within organizations, such as government agencies, corporations, and educational institutions. They often maintain racial hierarchies and perpetuate biases and stereotypes. Examples of institutional practices include:

- Biased hiring and promotion practices.
- Racial profiling by law enforcement.
- Unequal disciplinary actions in schools.

These practices can contribute to the systemic marginalization and exclusion of racial minority groups.

Cultural representations and narratives also contribute to structural racism. Media, entertainment, and other cultural industries often reinforce stereotypes and biases, shaping public opinion and perpetuating racial inequities. Portrayals of racial minority groups as criminals, exotic or inferior, for instance, can contribute to the stigmatization and marginalization of these communities.

These representations shape societal attitudes and can influence policy decisions and individual behavior.

Structural racism is a self-perpetuating system deeply ingrained within society's institutions and practices. Its effects are far-reaching, leading to disparities in access to quality education, healthcare, employment opportunities, and wealth accumulation.

These disparities, in turn, reinforce and perpetuate existing racial inequities, creating a cycle of disadvantage for marginalized communities.

Addressing structural racism requires comprehensive and systemic change. It involves examining and challenging discriminatory policies, implementing equitable practices within institutions, and promoting inclusive cultural representations.

Additionally, it requires acknowledging historical injustices, engaging in meaningful dialogue, and actively working to dismantle the structures and systems that perpetuate racial inequities.

Efforts to combat structural racism often involve:

- Advocating for policy reforms.

- Implementing diversity and inclusion initiatives.

- Supporting community-led initiatives.

- Promoting anti-racist education.

By addressing the root causes of racial inequity and working towards systemic change, societies can begin to dismantle the structures that perpetuate structural racism and strive toward a more equitable and just future for all.

Although, that wouldn't be enough to justify the stand of equity against racism. We would have to go down history lane — where racial scrutiny began and understand its roots in other to cut down the now bloomed tree of unjust.

Historical context

Here is an exploration of the historical aspects of racial discrimination in America, focusing on the healthcare system and reproductive rights, along with notable events, policies, and legislation that have influenced the experiences of black women during pregnancy and childbirth:

1. Slavery and Medical Experimentation: During the era of slavery, black women were subjected to medical experimentation without their consent or consideration for their well-being. Enslaved black women were used as subjects for experiments in gynecology, obstetrics, and surgical procedures, contributing to a long history of medical exploitation and trauma.

2. Jim Crow Era: During the Jim Crow era, racial segregation and discriminatory practices permeated the healthcare system. Black women faced limited access to quality healthcare facilities and often had to rely on under-resourced and segregated institutions that provided substandard care.

3. Forced Sterilisation: In the mid-20th century, black women were disproportionately targeted for forced sterilization procedures, often without informed consent. This practice, known as eugenics, aimed to control the population of marginalized communities and was enforced through policies and medical practices.

4. The "Mississippi Appendectomy": In the mid-20th century, black women in the South were victims of a practice known as the "Mississippi Appendectomy." This term referred to the forced sterilization of black women during other medical procedures, such as cesarean sections or appendectomies, without their knowledge or consent.

5. The Hyde Amendment: In 1976, the Hyde Amendment was passed, restricting federal funding for abortion services. This policy disproportionately affected low-income women, including many black women, limiting their access to safe and affordable reproductive healthcare.

6. Maternal Mortality and Morbidity Crisis: Black women in America face significantly higher maternal mortality and morbidity rates than their white counterparts. The historical lack of access to quality healthcare, racial biases, and systemic disparities contribute to this crisis, highlighting the persistent racial discrimination in maternal healthcare.

7. The Affordable Care Act (ACA): The ACA, passed in 2010, aimed to improve access to healthcare for millions of Americans. It included provisions to address disparities in maternal health and improve coverage for prenatal care. However, challenges remain in fully addressing the racial disparities in maternal healthcare.

8. The Black Maternal Health Omnibus Act: Introduced in 2021, the Black Maternal Health Omnibus Act is a comprehensive package of legislation addressing the maternal health crisis in the United States, focusing on black women.

The bill includes provisions to invest in community-based organizations, improve maternal healthcare data collection, expand Medicaid coverage, and support innovative approaches to maternity care.

By examining these historical events, policies, and legislation, we can better understand the systemic nature of racial discrimination in the healthcare system and reproductive rights in America. This historical context underscores the need for ongoing efforts to address these disparities and ensure equitable access to quality care for all women, regardless of their racial or ethnic background.

Now back to my story! I knew something was off with the doctors, so I got a new one. I had an appointment scheduled in June to see a new doctor, and to my surprise, there was a change in the on-duty physician. Now, a lady was taking care of me. She insisted on running more tests, even though I told her I felt excellent with no complaints. I questioned the need for these additional tests, and she explained that it was a routine procedure for the baby's well-being. Reluctantly, I agreed.

Chapter Four

Unveiling the Invisible: My Encounter with Racial Bias in Obstetric Care

I remembered a previous incident at the lab where they struggled to draw blood from me. After a few tubes, they realized no blood was flowing and attributed it to my dehydration. In June, I received a call from the clinic on a Monday morning.

The lady informed me that my liver enzymes test had returned with high levels. This news hit me like a ton of bricks. She said I needed to schedule two more appointments, one for an X-ray and another to see an oncologist. I suggested doing the X-ray before jumping to conclusions about seeing an oncologist. I was confident the other tests they had asked me to do wouldn't reveal anything worrisome. However, the doctor herself called me to insist on proceeding with all the tests. I couldn't help but wonder why she had tested my liver when I had no complaints and the focus was supposed to be on the baby.

Fear, anger, and anxiety consumed me at that moment. What if I had preeclampsia, kidney stones, or liver problems? I had two children, ages 11 and 7, relying on me for their well-being. It was time to change my doctor and seek a fresh start.

I registered at another hospital, Grady, where I gave birth to my second child without complications or headaches. At this point, I was filled with anger, frustration, and fear. What if my health was in serious jeopardy? What if I genuinely had all these medical issues?

My mind was spinning with worries as I went to the hospital, arriving a bit late at around 4:30 pm. They could only accommodate me at the emergency department, and I would have to return for my prenatal clinic appointment. I accepted this arrangement, as it was better than nothing. Surprisingly, my blood pressure during pregnancy was 130/75, which is considered relatively normal. The news I received within six weeks of joining that previous doctor's hospital had been overwhelming and disheartening.

I had only seen two of their doctors so far, and they had already bombarded me with bad news. I was told I would meet with their doctors before the delivery, ensuring that any of them on duty at the bigger hospital could deliver my baby.

Returning to Grady felt familiar, as I had been here before when I gave birth to my second child. I remembered how the nurses would introduce me to the doctors, highlighting that I was a 32-year-old female with perfect health.

Now, at 39 years old, nothing has changed. I was still not on any prescriptions and had gotten pregnant without trying. The memories of my previous smooth pregnancy filled my mind. I had been scheduled for a cesarean section after 40 weeks of not going into labor. As I waited to be seen by the doctor at Grady, I yearned for a change in my medical care. I wanted to switch doctors and voiced my concerns about the high liver enzyme levels I had been told about. The doctor asked if I had complained about anything before the liver test, and I honestly replied with a no. She assured me that doctors don't just run tests casually. She looked at me and said, "Doctors don't just run tests on you for no reason."

She then examined me. I lay on the examination table as she carefully read me, pointing out where my liver was. I had no idea until that moment. With a smile, she uttered those reassuring words I longed to hear, "Everything looks good.

You have perfect health." With that, she discharged me, promising someone would call me soon to schedule my prenatal appointments. Before leaving, I signed a form to transfer my medical records from my previous doctor's office.

As I made my way home, a whirlwind of thoughts raced through my mind. I have a 10-year-old boy and a 6-year-old girl who depend on me. The weight of responsibility pressed upon me, and I realized the need to secure life insurance to cover my debts and provide for my children's future in case something happened to me. I began to notice how I clung to my kids, hugging them tightly, and how I found myself sneaking into their rooms at night, just watching them sleep. The uncertainty gnawed at me, and I couldn't help but ponder who would care for them if the worst were to occur.

Nights were the hardest. I would lie on my bed, tears streaming down my face, consumed by thoughts of what the doctor had said about my heart, kidneys, and liver—those vital organs that sustain our lives.

Determined to protect my children, I searched for life insurance. It became my lifeline, my shield against an uncertain future. My children were my world, and I vowed to ensure their well-being no matter what.

In contemplating guardianship, I considered entrusting my estate to my older brother, a wise economist with a knack for managing finances. I knew he would ensure my children's financial security.

Another option was my sister-in-law, my brother's wife, who possessed a sweet and caring soul and legal expertise as a lawyer. She would undoubtedly provide love and support to my children. Then there was my only blood sister, though she resided in Ireland. I wanted to know if my kids would be open to moving to a different country and experiencing a new culture and way of life.

These thoughts consumed me as I walked the path of uncertainty, but my children remained my beacon of hope through it all. I resolved to protect them, secure their future, and cherish every moment spent together. They were my reason for being, the very essence of my existence.

There has to be a way to counter this disturbing factor in the lives of pregnant black women in America. This leads back to structural racism and its Effect on black women's lives.

Chapter Five

The Intersection of Racism and Maternal Mortality

More On Structural Racism (in-depth knowledge)

Structural racism is a deeply ingrained and systemic issue affecting various societal aspects, perpetuating racial inequalities and injustices. It refers to how social, economic, and political systems are designed to create and maintain advantages for specific racial or ethnic groups while disadvantaging others.

Unlike individual acts of racism based on personal beliefs and actions, structural racism operates at a broader level, embedded within institutions, policies, and practices.

One key aspect of structural racism is the historical legacy of discrimination and oppression that has disproportionately impacted marginalized communities, particularly people of color. Centuries of slavery, segregation, and discriminatory policies have left a lasting impact on the social and economic conditions faced by racial minority groups.

These historical injustices have led to disparities in education, housing, employment, healthcare, and criminal justice. Structural racism manifests in various ways.

It can be seen in policies and practices perpetuating racial disparities, such as discriminatory housing practices limiting access to safe and affordable housing for people of color or discriminatory hiring practices restricting employment opportunities.

It can also be observed in the unequal distribution of resources, such as disparities in educational funding that perpetuate gaps in quality education between predominantly white and minority communities.

In addition to institutional biases, cultural representations and media portrayals often reinforce stereotypes and prejudices, further contributing to the perpetuation of structural racism. These representations shape public perceptions and can influence decision-making processes that perpetuate inequalities.

Addressing structural racism requires a multi-faceted approach. It involves recognizing and acknowledging the historical and ongoing systemic injustices marginalized communities face. It also entails implementing policies and practices that actively dismantle these inequalities and create equitable opportunities for all individuals, regardless of their racial or ethnic background.

Efforts to address structural racism include advocating for policies that promote equal access to education, healthcare, employment, and housing. It involves promoting diversity, inclusion, and representation within institutions and decision-making bodies.

Additionally, initiatives aimed at raising awareness, promoting dialogue, and fostering understanding about the impacts of structural racism are crucial for building a more equitable and just society.

Ultimately, combating structural racism requires a collective commitment to dismantling systemic barriers and creating a society where individuals are not limited by their racial or ethnic background but have equal opportunities to thrive and succeed.

In the United States, African Americans face unique challenges regarding the health of mothers and babies. Factors like income, education, and social status, which usually protect white Americans, don't offer the same protection for African Americans.

These factors are known as social determinants of health, including where people live, work, and play. Unfortunately, racism is a significant part of being black in America, and it directly affects the health of African American women and their infants. We need to look at this urgent public health crisis through a lens of racial justice.

Structural racism is a system where policies, practices, and cultural norms work together to maintain racial inequality. It's powered by primarily white people in positions of authority who contribute to these imbalances. To address the maternal and infant mortality crisis, we must use social justice frameworks that intentionally tackle these power imbalances. One such framework is called reproductive justice. It focuses on women's rights, especially women of color, to have complete control over their bodies and to parent with dignity.

Reproductive justice recognizes that a woman's ability to make decisions about her reproductive health is influenced by the conditions in her community, such as access to healthcare, affordable housing, and economic opportunities. Therefore, policy solutions must prioritize communities of color and consider their specific needs to address the racial disparities in maternal and infant mortality effectively.

Racism in healthcare can take on various forms, and its effects are not limited to individual biases. It can be seen in the unequal distribution of quality healthcare facilities and providers in communities predominantly consisting of people of color.

Additionally, these communities often face harsh environmental conditions and exposure to toxins, particularly in African American neighborhoods. The workplace inequalities, concentrated food insecurity, and policy changes targeting healthcare programs like Medicaid further exacerbate the disparities faced by people of color.

It's essential to recognize that biases related to other social factors, such as education, income, sexual orientation, disability, and immigration status, can also harm patients' experiences and health outcomes within healthcare settings. Moreover, the intersection of racism and sexism adds another layer of discrimination, particularly affecting women of color.

African American, Latina, AIAN (American Indian, Alaska Native), and Asian and Pacific Islander women consistently face bias and discrimination based on their race and gender when seeking healthcare. This compounded discrimination often leaves women, especially women of color, feeling invisible and unheard when seeking medical assistance or expressing concerns about pain and discomfort during and after childbirth.

In essence, the far-reaching effects of racism in healthcare go beyond individual biases, affecting access to care, environmental conditions, workplace dynamics, food security, policy changes, and the intersectional experiences of women of color. It is crucial to address these issues to ensure equitable and inclusive healthcare for all.

Extensive evidence highlights the detrimental effects of racism on African American women's mental, emotional, and physical health throughout their lives. However, it is crucial to recognize that racism doesn't just impact individuals; it also affects the health of their infants and families.

Health disparities in maternal and infant health conditions, such as maternal mental health, sudden infant death syndrome (SIDS), sudden unexpected infant deaths (SUID), and cesarean section deliveries, shed light on how structural racism and bias can influence health outcomes.

SIDS/SUID is a leading cause of infant mortality in the United States, and higher rates of cesarean section deliveries are associated with increased maternal mortality and severe maternal morbidity.

It is concerning that in 2017, the rate of C-sections among black women was 36 percent, compared to 30.9 percent among non-Hispanic white women. Additionally, in 2013, the SIDS/SUID rate for black women was approximately twice as high as that of non-Hispanic white women. These disparities can be attributed, in part, to factors such as underinsurance, limited access to quality maternity and neonatal care facilities, and the scarcity of hospitals in underserved communities.

By understanding these disparities and their underlying causes, we can gain insight into the urgent need for addressing structural racism and bias within the healthcare system. It is essential to promote equal access to quality care for African American women and their families, as this will positively impact their overall health and well-being.

The following sections present policy recommendations to tackle structural racism within the healthcare and family support systems. These recommendations are designed to address the root causes of racial disparities and provide enhanced support and services to pregnant women and new mothers, mitigating the adverse effects of racism on their experiences.

It is crucial to acknowledge racism as the fundamental factor contributing to maternal and infant deaths to develop effective policy solutions that can eliminate racial inequalities. To ensure a comprehensive approach that considers the historical and ongoing impact of racism, policy solutions should adopt a targeted universalism approach.

This equity framework combines targeted strategies to achieve a universal goal, ensuring that policy solutions cater to the needs of all populations while intentionally prioritizing the most vulnerable group—African American women and families.

The following are the above-stated recommendations for tackling structural racism:

Strengthen existing health programs and support reproductive health care

The topic emphasizes the importance of strengthening existing health programs and supporting reproductive health care, particularly for women. Policymakers are urged to focus on bolstering critical components of the healthcare system, such as Medicaid, the Affordable Care Act (ACA), and the Children's Health Insurance Program (CHIP), which provide coverage to millions of women and their children.

Comprehensive and affordable healthcare coverage is essential for women throughout their lives but becomes particularly crucial during pregnancy and postnatal. Access to adequate maternity care and healthcare coverage has significant and lasting positive impacts on the mother and her child.

Women lacking health care coverage may be compelled to forgo routine prenatal and postnatal care, which is vital for identifying health risks and preventing complications.

Reports from maternal mortality review committees (MMRCs) collaborating with the Centers for Disease Control and Prevention (CDC) Foundation reveal that approximately 60 percent of maternal deaths are preventable. This statistic underscores the urgent need to prioritize accessible and comprehensive health care for pregnant women.

Furthermore, focusing on preventing common conditions associated with maternal mortality can have a significant impact. For instance, cardiovascular and coronary diseases are reported to be 68 percent preventable, while hemorrhage is 70 percent preventable. These figures demonstrate the potential for reducing maternal mortality rates through improved access to reproductive health care and comprehensive coverage.

By strengthening health programs like Medicaid, the ACA, and CHIP, policymakers can ensure women have the resources to obtain quality prenatal and postnatal care.

These programs can help provide essential services, such as regular check-ups, screenings, and interventions to manage potential complications. By supporting reproductive health care, policymakers can contribute to healthier pregnancies, safer childbirths, and improved outcomes for women and their children.

In summary, prioritizing strengthening existing health programs and supporting reproductive health care is crucial for the well-being of women. By focusing on comprehensive coverage and accessibility, policymakers can address preventable maternal mortality and promote positive health outcomes for women throughout their reproductive years.

Expanding Agencies like Medicaid in All States.

These services are like superhero sidekicks for mothers and infants, swooping in to provide crucial support when it matters most. Imagine a dynamic duo fighting the villains of health risks and ensuring a happy and healthy journey through pregnancy and beyond.

First, we have the mighty Management of Chronic Disease, armed with the power to keep women in continuous treatment. With this force, mothers can minimize these conditions' risks throughout their pregnancy and even afterward. It's like having a trusty guardian angel watching over them, ensuring they receive the care they need.

Next, we have incredible Access to Contraception, the ultimate defender against unplanned and high-risk pregnancies. Their powers help women avoid the unexpected and make well-informed choices. They're like a reliable shield, protecting against the perils of unintended pregnancies.

And let's not forget about the invincible Pregnancy and Maternal Care coverage! With this superpower, women can access the care they need, ensuring a safer journey for themselves and their little ones. This coverage has been proven to lower the risk factors associated with low birth weight and early-term births. It's like having a magical cloak that shields against potential health hazards.

When these three powers unite, they create a comprehensive healthcare force that can work wonders. They can significantly improve women's health before and during pregnancy, tremendously impacting infant mortality rates. It's like assembling an unstoppable team that tackles the challenges head-on.

But wait, there's more! Research has shown that Medicaid expansion is a true lifesaver. According to a study in the American Journal of Public Health, states that expanded Medicaid saw a decline in infant mortality rates, with the most significant reduction among African American infants. That's like a victory dance for justice and equality!

The Center for American Progress estimates that expanding Medicaid in non-expansion states could save the lives of 141 infants each year. It's like a powerful potion that brings hope and better health outcomes to those who most need it.

Sadly, in some states, restrictions and eligibility hurdles prevent pregnant women and new mothers from enjoying the full benefits of healthcare coverage. But fear not! Federal law should require states to extend the range for new mothers beyond the current 60-day postpartum period, at least up to one year after giving birth.

This brave move would ensure that mothers receive the care they need during this critical time. It's like a magical spell that grants access to comprehensive healthcare to those who deserve it.

And let's remember our superheroines of color! This extension of care would be a game-changer, providing health and economic benefits to new mothers from diverse backgrounds.

Since women of color are more likely to be covered by Medicaid, an essential program that supports nearly half of all births in the United States, it becomes a vital tool in tackling racial disparities in maternal and infant mortality. It's like a beacon of hope, shining a light on equality and fairness for all.

So, let's join forces and celebrate the triumphs of these fantastic services. They may not wear capes, but they possess the power to change lives, saving mothers and infants from the clutches of health risks and disparities. Together, we can build a healthier and happier future for everyone!

Eliminate maternity care deserts.

Access to maternity care is a significant issue in rural and urban areas, particularly for African American and low-income families. A recent study revealed that over half of rural counties lack obstetric services, and these services are even scarcer in rural counties with higher populations of African American and low-income families. Additionally, the closure of maternity wards primarily serving African American residents in Washington, D.C., has severely limited women's access to maternity care.

Unfortunately, the problem of limited access to quality care is not exclusive to rural settings. Women of color, particularly in urban areas, face disparities in receiving high-quality obstetric care and are more likely to deliver in lower-quality hospitals. These disparities contribute to poorer health outcomes for both mothers and infants.

The closure of hospitals, including obstetric wards, has exacerbated the issue by increasing the distance women must travel for maternity care.

This situation disproportionately affects low-income women and women of color, creating additional barriers to access and increasing their risk. Research has shown that traveling long distances for healthcare negatively impacts outcomes and threatens the lives of women and infants.

Policymakers should fully enforce the Improving Access to Maternity Care Act (Public Law No: 115-320) enacted in December 2018 to address these challenges and eliminate maternity care deserts.

This law mandates the Health Resources and Services Administration (HRSA), an agency within the U.S. Department of Health and Human Services (HHS), to identify and gather data on areas experiencing a shortage of maternity care professionals.

Additionally, policymakers should direct the HRSA to share best practices and lessons learned from existing programs, such as the Remote Pregnancy Monitoring Challenge.

These initiatives leverage technology to enhance access to care in low-income rural and urban settings, aiming to inform the development of effective care models for pregnant women in these areas.

Identifying maternity care deserts is vital for the HRSA and the National Health Service Corps (NHSC). The NHSC is crucial in addressing workforce shortages in underserved areas by implementing recruitment efforts, scholarships, and loan repayment programs for healthcare professionals like physicians, nurse practitioners, certified nurse midwives, and physician assistants.

By prioritizing the enforcement of existing legislation, sharing best practices, and leveraging technology, policymakers can make significant strides in improving access to maternity care for all women, especially black women, throughout the United States.

Offer African American women tools to navigate health settings.

Empowering African American women with a splendid array of birthing options and top-notch prenatal care can sprinkle their journey to motherhood with extra magic, resulting in positive birth experiences and healthy pregnancies.

While some state Medicaid programs offer a taste of midwifery care, it's high time to turn up the volume and fully immerse these enchanting services into state health systems.

Let's cast a spell to expand insurance coverage for doula services, ensuring that every expectant mother can access these invaluable support systems regardless of her insurance or income level. We're on a quest to unlock the treasure trove of birthing choices and reproductive autonomy for low-income women and women of color!

Imagine a world where doulas, the mystical guides of motherhood, stand by every pregnant woman's side, providing gentle whispers of encouragement and soothing potions of comfort. Picture midwives, the guardians of natural birthing wisdom, joining forces with modern medicine, creating a harmonious blend of tradition and innovation. Together, they create a symphony of care that echoes through every community, embracing diversity and celebrating the unique stories of each woman.

But that's not all! We must also wield the power of health literacy and education to equip African American women with the knowledge and confidence to navigate the labyrinth of healthcare decisions. Let's unlock the secrets of wellness, unraveling the mysteries of pregnancy and childbirth so that every mother can hold the reins of her destiny.

With these enchanting transformations, we can paint a vibrant tapestry where every expectant mother feels like the queen of her fairy tale, empowered to make choices that align with her values and aspirations. Together, we will dance to the rhythm of healthier pregnancies, joyful births, and flourishing families to create a realm where every woman's dreams become a reality.

One way to increase access to midwives and ensure high-quality maternity care is through integrating midwifery care with primary health care. A study conducted by the Birth Place Lab in the Division of Midwifery at the University of British Columbia found that for states with integrated midwifery care throughout health care systems, families were more likely to have full access to high-quality maternity care.

The study conceptualized integration as the ability of midwives to work entirely in the scope of their practice autonomously and without unnecessary restrictions within both traditional (hospitals) and nontraditional health settings (birthing centers and home births).

This work was done collaboratively with other healthcare professionals. Washington State, New Mexico, and Oregon were ranked highest for integration. The states cited as being hostile to midwives were concentrated in the South and had large African American populations.

In addition to coverage expansions and easing restrictive laws and regulations on the practice of midwifery, policymakers should do more to fully integrate both midwifery care and doula services in health systems, which could be particularly impactful in states with large African American populations or within states with high rates of maternal and infant mortality. Better integration could be achieved by ensuring the availability of skilled doulas and midwives in hospitals and birthing centers, focusing on doulas and midwives of color, and ensuring close coordination and collaborative working partnerships with nurses and OB-GYNs.

Private Insurance Plans Should Cover Doula And Doula Services

Private insurance plans often need to consistently cover midwifery and doula services, mainly if they are provided outside of hospital settings. While most insurers usually cover certified nurse-midwives (CNMs), only six states have laws in place that require private insurance to cover certified professional midwives (CPMs) who work in birthing centers and home births.

This means that many mothers and families have to bear the expensive costs of doula care out of their own pockets, as private insurance coverage for doulas is not mandated in any state.

Furthermore, coverage for birthing centers varies greatly among private insurance plans. While Medicaid is required to provide coverage for licensed birth centers under the Affordable Care Act (ACA), private insurers do not have the same obligation. Consequently, the availability of range for these services and the number of in-network providers for non-hospital maternity care differ significantly depending on the private insurance plan and the insurer. It's a complex landscape where the support and choices for expectant mothers can vary dramatically.

Increase the range of birth options.

Increasing the range of birth options is vital in addressing structural racism in healthcare. Structural racism refers to the systemic and institutionalized policies, practices, and beliefs perpetuating racial inequalities. In the context of birth options, it refers to the disparities and inequities experienced by marginalized communities, particularly people of color, during pregnancy, childbirth, and postpartum care.

Expanding birth options can help counter structural racism by providing greater autonomy, choice, and access to culturally appropriate care for expectant parents. Here are some ways in which increases the range of birth options can address structural racism:

1. Diverse birthing settings: Offering a diverse range of birthing settings, such as hospitals, birth centers, and home births, can provide options that align with individuals' preferences, cultural practices, and comfort levels. Some communities have cultural traditions and practices that are better supported in non-hospital settings, and providing access to such options can improve birth outcomes and experiences.

2. Midwifery care: Expanding access to midwifery care, particularly by increasing the number of midwives from diverse backgrounds, can help address racial disparities in maternal and infant health outcomes. Research has shown that midwifery care, which emphasizes holistic, patient-centered, and culturally sensitive approaches, can improve outcomes for communities facing systemic racism and discrimination.

3. Doula support: Doulas are trained professionals who provide emotional, physical, and informational support to individuals during pregnancy, childbirth, and postpartum. Increasing access to doula services, particularly for marginalized communities, can improve birth experiences, reduce maternal complications, and mitigate the effects of racism and bias within healthcare systems.

4. Culturally competent care: Healthcare providers need to be culturally competent and sensitive to the needs and experiences of diverse populations. Training healthcare professionals to address implicit biases, understand cultural practices, and communicate effectively with patients from different backgrounds is essential for reducing racial disparities in birth outcomes.

5. Community-led initiatives: Encouraging community-led initiatives that provide support and resources for expectant parents can empower marginalized communities and address structural racism. These initiatives may involve community health workers, grassroots organizations, or partnerships between healthcare providers and community leaders to ensure culturally appropriate care and support.

6. Advocacy and policy changes: Addressing structural racism requires advocacy for policy changes at the local, state, and national levels. Advocacy efforts can focus on improving reimbursement policies to increase access to non-hospital birth options, supporting the diversification of the healthcare workforce, and promoting equitable funding for maternal and infant healthcare.

In conclusion, expanding the range of birth options can help counter structural racism by providing expectant parents with greater autonomy, choice, and access to culturally appropriate care. By addressing racial disparities in healthcare and ensuring equitable access to quality care, we can work towards a more just and inclusive healthcare system for all individuals, regardless of their racial or ethnic background.

Halt the overuse of C-sections in the United States.

In the United States, there is a growing concern about the excessive use of Caesarean sections (C-sections) during childbirth.

Recent research has shown that providing prenatal education and support through trained doulas to a diverse group of Medicaid recipients can help reduce the likelihood of C-sections and preterm births. This finding holds even after considering various clinical and socio-demographic factors.

A C-section is a surgical procedure where the baby is delivered through an incision in the mother's abdomen and uterus. Compared to vaginal deliveries, C-sections are associated with higher risks. These risks include potential injuries to the baby during surgery, infections, excessive bleeding after birth, blood clots, and increased complications in future pregnancies. The rates of maternal mortality and severe maternal health issues are approximately three times higher for women undergoing C-sections than those with vaginal deliveries.

Unfortunately, there is a disparity in C-section rates among different racial and ethnic groups in the United States. Black women, even with low-risk pregnancies, are more likely to undergo C-sections compared to other women of color groups and white women. This disparity is particularly evident in states like Louisiana, Mississippi, and Florida, where the percentage of African American residents is high, and C-section rates exceed 37 percent.

To address this issue, it is crucial to focus on reducing the overuse of C-sections in the United States. Providing prenatal education and support, mainly through trained doulas, can significantly lower C-section rates and promote healthier outcomes for mothers and babies. Additionally, efforts should be made to address the racial disparities in C-section rates, ensuring that all women, regardless of ethnicity, receive appropriate and evidence-based care during childbirth.

Indeed, studies have shown that black women in the United States experience disproportionately high cesarean section (C-section) delivery rates compared to women of other racial and ethnic backgrounds. This disparity in C-section rates is a concerning issue highlighting racial and healthcare inequities within the country.

Multiple factors contribute to the higher C-section rates among black women. One significant factor is racial bias and systemic racism within the healthcare system.

Research has found that black women are more likely to be subjected to medical interventions, including C-sections, even when they have similar health profiles and medical needs as white women. This racial bias can stem from stereotypes, implicit biases, and unequal treatment, leading to unnecessary medical interventions.

Another contributing factor is the higher prevalence of certain health conditions among black women, such as obesity, hypertension, and diabetes, which can increase the likelihood of complications during pregnancy and necessitate a C-section. Socioeconomic factors, including limited access to quality healthcare, lower socioeconomic status, and higher poverty rates, also affect the higher C-section rates among black women.

Moreover, a lack of culturally competent care and inadequate communication between healthcare providers and black women can further contribute to the disparity. Research has shown that black women often face dismissive attitudes, lack of respect, and inadequate information from healthcare professionals, resulting in a less favorable birth experience and a higher likelihood of C-sections.

The consequences of the disproportionately high C-section rates for black women are significant. C-sections carry their risks and complications, including longer recovery times, increased risk of infection, and potential difficulties in subsequent pregnancies. Additionally, the emotional and psychological impact of an unwanted or medically unnecessary C-section can be substantial.

Addressing and reducing the disparities in C-section rates among black women require a multifaceted approach. Healthcare providers and institutions must undergo cultural sensitivity training and work to eliminate racial bias in decision-making processes. Increasing access to quality prenatal care and education for black women can help manage health conditions and reduce the need for interventions. Policymakers must prioritize initiatives that address healthcare inequities and promote equitable access to comprehensive reproductive healthcare services.

In conclusion, the disproportionately high C-section rates among black women in the United States reflect racial and healthcare inequities. Addressing this disparity necessitates systemic changes, including addressing racial bias, improving cultural competence in healthcare, increasing access to quality prenatal care, and advocating for policies that promote equitable healthcare for all women, regardless of their racial or ethnic background.

Ensure health literacy and childbirth education.

Policymakers must prioritize grant funding for health literacy, education, and training specifically tailored to address the needs of black American women. This support is crucial to sustain and expand vital programs led by community-based organizations led by black American women. Additionally, this funding can facilitate the assessment and evaluation of these programs and their replication and adaptation for broader communities and audiences. Policymakers and public agencies should take the lead in driving significant changes within the current healthcare system and challenging traditional practices perpetuating racial discrimination against black American women.

This includes the development of policies, guidelines, and regulations that empower healthcare providers to combat persistent disparities actively. Moreover, policymakers should encourage practitioners to form partnerships beyond the conventional health and educational sectors, enabling them to engage and serve their patients and clients effectively.

Improve the quality of care provided to black pregnant women.

Improving the quality of care provided to pregnant Black American women is essential to addressing racial disparities in maternal health outcomes. Black women in the United States experience disproportionately higher maternal mortality and morbidity rates than their white counterparts. This disparity is often attributed to socioeconomic, systemic, and racial factors, including implicit bias, structural racism, and barriers to accessing high-quality healthcare. To address these disparities and enhance the quality of care, several key areas should be considered:

1. Cultural Competency and Anti-Bias Training: Healthcare providers should receive cultural competency and anti-bias training to understand the unique experiences and challenges Black American women face. This training can help mitigate implicit biases and stereotypes that may impact the quality of care provided.

2. Addressing Implicit Bias: Healthcare institutions must implement strategies to identify and address implicit bias within their systems. This can involve standardized protocols and guidelines that promote equitable treatment and decision-making and regular assessments and feedback mechanisms to monitor and correct biases.

3. Enhancing Prenatal Care: Care should be comprehensive, accessible, and culturally sensitive. This includes providing early and consistent prenatal care, addressing social determinants of health such as poverty and housing instability, and offering personalized care plans that consider Black American women's specific needs and preferences.

4. Health Education and Outreach: Community-based health education programs should be developed to empower Black American women with information about pregnancy, childbirth, and postpartum care. These programs should address common myths, misconceptions, and cultural beliefs that may hinder access to quality care.

5. Diversifying the Healthcare Workforce: Increasing diversity within the healthcare workforce, including physicians, nurses, midwives, and doulas, is crucial. Having more Black healthcare professionals can help foster trust, improve communication, and provide culturally competent care that better aligns with the experiences and needs of Black American women.

6. Engaging Community Organisations: Collaboration with community-based organizations, such as doulas, midwifery groups, and advocacy organizations, is essential for providing holistic support to pregnant Black American women. These partnerships can help bridge gaps in access to care, provide emotional support, and advocate for policy changes that address systemic issues.

7. Data Collection and Research: Collecting accurate and comprehensive data on racial disparities in maternal health outcomes is crucial. This data can help identify specific areas where the quality of care needs improvement, inform evidence-based interventions, and monitor progress over time.

8. Policy Changes and Advocacy: Advocacy efforts should be directed towards implementing policies that address systemic racism and healthcare inequities. This includes policies that expand Medicaid coverage, improve access to affordable healthcare, promote reimbursement for doula services, and support initiatives that reduce racial disparities in maternal health outcomes.

Improving the quality of care for pregnant Black American women requires a multifaceted approach that addresses individual and systemic factors. By implementing these strategies, healthcare systems can significantly reduce racial disparities and ensure equitable and quality care for all pregnant women, regardless of race or ethnicity.

Train providers to address racism and build a more diverse healthcare workforce

To enhance cultural humility among healthcare professionals, it is crucial to incorporate a service-learning component into their training. This component would involve physicians and nurses working in underserved communities, enabling them to understand their patients' lived experiences better.

Additionally, it is essential to address and dismantle perceptions about biological differences between racial groups, especially those that perpetuate stereotypes about African Americans, such as the notion that they have "tougher skin."

To ensure the effectiveness of cultural humility training, they should be regularly assessed and evaluated by state and local health departments. This evaluation process can involve patient surveys and interviews to gather feedback and insights. By collecting this data over time, policymakers can utilize the results as part of broader initiatives to align payment with quality healthcare. This may involve rewarding healthcare providers who successfully reduce racial disparities in maternal and infant mortality, thus incentivizing the delivery of equitable care.

Chapter Six

Breaking the Silence: Sharing My Struggles with Racism in Pregnancy

There's still a lot where that came from, but not to bore you, allow me to return to my story. Please don't bother; it didn't get a sad ending like most tragic stories. This is my real-life experience, and I want the world to know. I would have loved to write this notice on Mother's Day, but I got caught up with work.

Well, here it is now, before you, the story of my third pregnancy and the difference between the previous pregnancy. As I sit here, reflecting on my journey of motherhood and the transformation I experienced during my third pregnancy, I am reminded of the unique challenges that many Black American women face in their motherhood journeys. It is essential to acknowledge that racial discrimination and disparities exist within the healthcare system, and they often disproportionately affect Black women, including during pregnancy and childbirth.

Black women in America are more likely to experience maternal mortality and morbidity rates that are significantly higher than those of their white counterparts. They often face disparities in access to quality prenatal care, higher rates of preterm births, and increased complications during childbirth. These disparities are rooted in systemic racism, implicit biases, and socioeconomic factors that impact Black communities.

Just as I found strength in vulnerability and sought support during my pregnancy, it is crucial to recognize that Black women also need adequate help, understanding, and resources throughout their motherhood journeys. By sharing stories and experiences, we can create awareness, advocate for change, and work towards dismantling the systemic barriers contributing to racial disparities in maternal healthcare.

I hope my story serves as a reminder of the resilience and power of self-discovery that can be found within all mothers, including Black American women. By celebrating the transformative nature of motherhood, we can also strive for a future where all mothers, regardless of race or ethnicity, receive equitable care and support, ensuring healthier outcomes for themselves and their children.

In solidarity with all mothers, particularly Black American women, let us continue to raise our voices, challenge the injustices, and work towards a society that embraces and celebrates the diversity and strength of motherhood.

I sat nervously in the waiting room, flipping through a magazine as I awaited my prenatal appointment at Grady. Being pregnant always brought excitement and anxiety, and today was no different. I had an important task on my mind – writing a will to ensure the well-being of my child, especially in case something unexpected happened to me. It was a responsibility I wanted to fulfill as a loving and caring parent.

As I sat there, thoughts of my sister crossed my mind. She was an incredible mother to her children, always putting their needs first and ensuring they were well cared for. I admired her dedication and hoped to be just as great of a mother to my child.

Finally, my name was called, and I followed the nurse to the examination room. The doctors soon entered, and I could sense a hint of curiosity in their eyes. They had read my medical notes from my previous doctors and were puzzled by their path regarding my blood pressure during pregnancy.

Based on my blood pressure readings, the new doctors reassured me there was no cause for alarm. They explained that they wouldn't have sent me for those tests because the tasks didn't indicate any issues. It was a relief to hear their professional opinion and to know that my health and my baby's health were not a cause for concern.

However, the doctors wanted to ensure a comprehensive understanding of my medical history, so they decided to run all the tests again. Four groups of doctors came into the room, each examining my records and discussing the situation amongst themselves. Their expressions seemed disappointed, perhaps because they had expected to find something alarming.

Nonetheless, they proceeded with the tests, conducting a thorough examination. I felt anxiety and hope as I waited for the results. Deep down, I knew that my body had been caring for me and my baby, but the uncertainty still lingered in my mind.

After what felt like an eternity, the doctors returned with the results. I held my breath as they delivered the news – everything was fine. There were no signs of high liver enzymes or kidney problems. My blood pressure remained stable, and my urine had no protein. A sigh of relief washed over me, knowing that my baby and I were healthy and thriving.

As I left the doctor's office that day, I couldn't help but feel an overwhelming sense of gratitude. I was grateful for the new doctors who reassured me and took the time to rerun the tests, even though they initially found no cause for concern. Their thoroughness brought me peace of mind and allowed me to focus on the joy and excitement of my pregnancy.

With the weight of worry lifted from my shoulders, I turned my attention back to the task of writing my will. As I contemplated the future, I was hopeful and determined to be the best mother I could be for my child. I knew that my sister's example and my love for my unborn baby would guide me through motherhood, no matter what challenges lay ahead.

Before I finish my experience with my third pregnancy, I wish to give more awareness and enlightenment on being pregnant and black in America or wherever you are as a colored person. I want to pour out as much public awareness on the racial scrutiny of black American women. And not just black women alone but every woman out there yet to have a baby, in the phase of having one or about to.

Continue reading and enjoy! The racial discriminated black American women aren't alone in this world! There are others like them out there in this world of unfairness. Being treated like they didn't pay taxes or like they living a free life without using money.

Yes, America isn't the only country where racism lies abreast without shame. You don't have to be necessarily black before you get looked down at. Merely being colored is enough to give you the stare of hate and disgust. This book should also serve as a remedy to every angle of this world where people cannot live freely because of the color of their skin. Or how they look, speak, eat or dance. It's only normal and beautiful that we look different from our neighbors. We all can't look the same, it would look just as absurd like a store of only white Lego toys. Where's the beauty in that? That wouldn't be fun, it wouldn't be beautiful either. Continue reading to get enlightened.

Racial Discrimination Against Black American Women: A Global Perspective.

Racial discrimination against black American women is not limited to the United States. Despite being a domestic concern, this issue extends beyond borders, affecting black women who travel, live, or work in other countries. This article aims to shed light on the experiences of black American women facing racial discrimination in various international contexts. It explores their challenges, the factors contributing to discrimination, and potential solutions.

1. Historical Context:

To understand the experiences of black American women facing discrimination abroad, it is crucial to examine the historical roots of racism and colonialism. Discuss the historical impact of the transatlantic slave trade, colonialism, and imperialism, which have shaped global power dynamics and influenced racial biases against black individuals.

2. Stereotypes and Prejudice:

Examine the stereotypes and prejudices black American women encounter in different countries. Explore how negative stereotypes perpetuated by media, culture, and historical narratives contribute to biased perceptions and discriminatory treatment. Address the intersectionality of race, gender, and nationality in shaping these stereotypes.

3. Employment Discrimination:

Discuss the challenges black American women face in accessing equal employment opportunities overseas. Analyze the systemic barriers, such as bias in hiring processes, limited career advancement prospects, and pay disparities. Explore case studies or research findings that highlight specific instances of discrimination in the workplace.

4. Educational Disparities:

Explore the educational disparities experienced by black American women studying or teaching abroad. Discuss how racial discrimination manifests within academic institutions, including biased admissions processes, limited support systems, and unequal resource access. Highlight initiatives that aim to address these disparities and promote inclusive educational environments.

5. Healthcare Disparities:

Examine the healthcare experiences of black American women living in foreign countries. Analyze the intersection of race, nationality, and gender in accessing quality healthcare, including challenges related to culturally competent care, language barriers, and biased medical practices. Discuss efforts to improve healthcare equity for Black American women in global healthcare systems.

6. Cultural Assimilation and Identity:

Discuss the complexities black American women face when navigating cultural assimilation in foreign countries. Explore the challenges of preserving their cultural identity while combating racial discrimination. Examine the intersection of race, nationality, and cultural dynamics and how it impacts the experiences of black American women abroad.

7. Activism and Advocacy:

Highlight the efforts of black American women and allies in fighting against racial discrimination on a global scale. Explore grassroots movements, advocacy organizations, and campaigns led by black American women to raise awareness, promote policy changes, and foster international solidarity against racism.

8. Legal Frameworks and International Human Rights:

Examine the legal frameworks and international human rights instruments that address racial discrimination. Discuss the role of international organizations, such as the United Nations, in advocating for the rights of black American women and combating racial discrimination globally.

9. Intersectionality and Allyship:

We have to analyze the importance of intersectionality in understanding the experiences of black American women facing discrimination abroad. Discuss the role of allyship in challenging racial discrimination and promoting inclusivity and equity. Highlight successful examples of intersectional allyship and collaborations in various countries.

10. Strategies for Change:

Provide recommendations and strategies to address racial discrimination faced by black American women abroad. Explore the importance of education, cultural exchange programs, policy changes, and international collaborations to combat discrimination. Discuss the role of individuals, communities, and governments in fostering a more inclusive and equitable global society.

Conclusion:

Racial discrimination against black American women is a complex issue beyond national boundaries. By understanding the experiences and challenges black American women face abroad, we can work towards dismantling systemic racism and promoting a more inclusive and equitable world. Through awareness, advocacy, and international cooperation, we can strive to create a future where racial scrutiny is abhorrent.

Chapter Seven

Advocating for Change: My Fight Against Racism in Maternal Healthcare

So I continued my prenatal care. I chose to have a cesarean section because I had my first two kids through c-sections. My cervix didn't open with my first boy, and my baby was already weighing over 9 pounds.

With my second child, I didn't even attempt a vaginal birth. I would have tried for the last one, but I was afraid of what my first doctors had told me. Throughout my pregnancy, I wasn't taking enough iron pills. The doctors at Grady Hospital gave me higher milligrams and suggested taking them with orange juice three times a day. My blood levels improved before delivery, and I had a healthy baby boy weighing 10 pounds and 6 ounces. I didn't experience any complications.

I am writing this book to raise awareness. If you are not comfortable with your doctors, please consider changing them. We know our bodies best. I hope this helps someone. We are sending love to all the mothers who didn't make it. We are black and proud, comfortable in our skin. We deserve to be treated equally as human beings, regardless of our race. We have families and people who depend on us.

A Comparative Analysis of Racial Discrimination Against Pregnant Black Women in America and Other Countries: Inspiring Change for an Equitable Future

Racial discrimination against pregnant black women is a distressing issue that transcends national borders. While acknowledging the gravity of this problem, it is vital to shed light on the experiences of black women in other countries where discrimination against them during pregnancy is prevalent. This article aims to compare and contrast the racial discrimination faced by pregnant black women in America with that experienced in other countries, emphasizing the urgency of addressing these issues. By appealing to the public's empathy and compassion, we can inspire change and work towards a more equitable future for all.

1. Understanding Racial Discrimination Against Pregnant Black Women:

Begin by providing a comprehensive overview of racial discrimination against pregnant black women in America. Discuss the historical context, social determinants, and structural factors contributing to this issue. Highlight the intersectionality of race and gender in shaping the experiences of black women during pregnancy.

2. Examining Other Countries with High Levels of Discrimination:

Identify several countries where racial discrimination against pregnant black women is prevalent. Select nations identified through research, international reports, or media coverage as having high levels of discrimination against black women during pregnancy. Offer an overview of each country's specific discriminatory practices or cultural biases.

3. Cultural Factors and Societal Attitudes:

Explore the cultural factors and societal attitudes that underpin racial discrimination against pregnant black women in the selected countries.

Discuss how historical legacies, cultural norms, and deeply entrenched biases contribute to discrimination and disparate treatment. Highlight specific examples or case studies to illustrate the impact of these factors on black women's experiences.

4. Legal and Policy Frameworks:

Compare the legal and policy frameworks in America and the selected countries that aim to address racial discrimination against pregnant black women. Evaluate these frameworks' effectiveness in protecting black women's rights and well-being during pregnancy. Discuss any gaps or limitations that hinder the enforcement of these laws and policies.

5. Health Disparities and Maternal Outcomes:

Analyze the health disparities and maternal outcomes for pregnant black women in America and the selected countries. Explore the impact of discrimination on access to prenatal care, quality of healthcare services, and maternal mortality rates. Highlight statistical data, research findings, and personal stories to illustrate black women's disparities in different healthcare systems.

6. Intersectionality and Multiple Forms of Discrimination:

Discuss the intersectionality of race, gender, and other identities in the experiences of pregnant black women. Explore how different forms of discrimination, such as socioeconomic status, immigrant status, or language barriers, intersect with racial discrimination to compound black women's challenges during pregnancy.

Emphasize the importance of an intersectional approach in addressing these complex issues.

7. Activism and Grassroots Movements:

Highlight the activism and grassroots movements led by black women and allies in America and the selected countries to combat pregnancy-related racial discrimination. Discuss the power of collective action, community organizing, and advocacy campaigns in raising awareness, promoting policy changes, and fostering societal transformation.

8. International Cooperation and Knowledge Exchange:

Explore the potential for international cooperation and knowledge exchange to address racial discrimination against pregnant black women. Discuss the importance of sharing best practices, research, and policy approaches between countries to facilitate a global movement for change. Highlight successful international collaborations and initiatives aimed at eradicating discrimination.

9. Media Representation and Public Awareness:

Examine the role of media representation in shaping public perception and raising awareness about racial discrimination against pregnant black women. Discuss the importance of accurate and balanced portrayals of black women's experiences in the media to challenge stereotypes and foster empathy. Explore the potential for storytelling, art, and other creative mediums to amplify the voices of black women and engage the public in the fight against discrimination.

10. Inspiring Change and Promoting Equity:

Conclude by emphasizing the importance of collective action and individual responsibility in combating racial discrimination against pregnant black women. Encourage readers to educate themselves, support advocacy organizations, and actively engage in efforts to promote equity and justice. Emphasize the transformative power of empathy, compassion, and solidarity in creating a more inclusive and equitable future for all.

Chapter Eight

Celebrating Resilience: Black Women's Strength in Overcoming Racial Challenges in Pregnancy

By comparing and contrasting the experiences of pregnant black women facing racial discrimination in America and other countries, we can foster a deeper understanding of this global issue. By appealing to the public's empathy and compassion, we have the potential to inspire meaningful change, challenge discriminatory practices, and work towards a future where every pregnant black woman receives equal respect, support, and care.

Embracing Empowerment and Advocacy: My Journey Towards a Healthy Caesarean Section

In this personal account, I share my transformative journey through three pregnancies, each leading to a cesarean section (CS) delivery. Past birth experiences, medical advice, and personal fears shaped my decisions.

Throughout my story, I aim to raise awareness about the importance of patient advocacy, the significance of seeking appropriate medical care, and the unique challenges black mothers-to-be face. By sharing my experiences, I hope to empower others to prioritize their well-being, challenge medical recommendations when necessary, and demand equitable treatment and care.

1. Birth Experiences and the Decision for Caesarean Sections:

My path into motherhood commenced with my first child, a son. Unfortunately, the delivery did not go as planned. My service provider failed to adequately monitor my progress, resulting in my and my baby's distress. With my second child, I opted for a scheduled CS as the fear of a repeat experience loomed.

For my third pregnancy, I contemplated a vaginal birth but succumbed to the fear instilled by my previous doctors. It became apparent that changes were necessary for the well-being of myself and my unborn child.

2. The Impact of Inadequate Prenatal Care and the Value of Iron Supplementation:

Throughout my pregnancies, I grappled with low iron levels. However, it was not until my third pregnancy, under the care of doctors at Grady, that the issue was addressed effectively. These healthcare professionals prescribed higher milligrams of iron supplements and recommended using orange juice thrice daily.

This proactive approach improved blood levels before delivery, ensuring a healthier pregnancy and minimizing the risk of complications during childbirth. This highlights the importance of comprehensive prenatal care and healthcare providers need to address individual needs.

3. Trusting Our Instincts and Advocating for Change:

My decision to undergo CS for my third child was partly influenced by the fear instilled in my previous birth experiences. Despite the potential benefits of attempting a vaginal birth after a cesarean (VBAC), I prioritize my mental and emotional well-being by avoiding unnecessary risks.

This experience underscored the importance of trusting our instincts as expectant mothers and advocating for our needs. It is crucial for black women, who face unique challenges within the healthcare system, to assert their rights to receive quality care free from discrimination or neglect.

4. The Significance of Changing Healthcare Providers:

One of the critical lessons I learned from my journey was the importance of finding healthcare providers who genuinely listen, respect, and prioritize the well-being of their patients.

As a black woman, I encountered biases and dismissive attitudes from some healthcare professionals. Through seeking care at Grady, I found doctors who understood my concerns, addressed my medical needs, and provided the support necessary for a successful CS. I strongly encourage others to advocate for themselves and change healthcare providers if they feel unheard or unsatisfied with the care they receive.

5. The Power of Sharing Experiences and Advocacy:

By sharing my story, I hope to raise awareness about the unique challenges black mothers-to-be face and inspire others to take control of their birthing experiences. It is crucial for expectant mothers to be proactive in their care, ask questions, and voice concerns to ensure their needs are met.

Additionally, I emphasize the significance of building a support network and seeking community resources to empower oneself and others. Together, we can challenge the status quo and demand equitable treatment.

Conclusion

My journey toward a healthy cesarean section has taught me the importance of patient advocacy, trust in one's instincts, and the pursuit of equitable care. Through my experiences, I have realized the power of sharing stories and raising awareness to inspire change.

Every expectant mother, regardless of race, deserves to be treated with respect, dignity, and equality. We must embrace empowerment and advocate for our rights within the healthcare system.

By amplifying our voices and demanding the care we deserve, we can create a world where all mothers can confidently embark on their birthing journeys, knowing that their well-being and the well-being of their babies are paramount.

Other key initiatives to ensure African American mothers and infants survive and thrive

1. Ensure workplace supports for pregnant women and new mothers

Supporting pregnant workers and new mothers in the workplace is crucial for ensuring their well-being and promoting positive health outcomes for both mothers and infants.

While several general measures can benefit all women, it is essential to recognize that African American women are often overrepresented in lower socioeconomic groups due to institutional racism. Addressing poverty and wealth inequality is critical in promoting reproductive justice and improving health outcomes for African American women and infants.

One key initiative is adopting a comprehensive national paid family and medical leave policy. Paid leave allows pregnant workers and new mothers to take time off to recover from childbirth, bond with their infants, and attend to their health needs. It provides financial stability and job security, which is particularly important for low-income women who may face additional financial burdens.

Ensuring access to high-quality and affordable childcare is another vital support for working mothers. Reasonable child care enables women to remain in the workforce while ensuring that their children receive appropriate care and early childhood education. This support is especially critical for low-income African American women who may struggle to access affordable childcare.

Enforcing and expanding the Pregnancy Discrimination Act (PDA) is essential for protecting the rights of pregnant workers. The PDA prohibits discrimination based on pregnancy, childbirth, or related medical conditions in employment. Ensuring that employers comply with these regulations and expanding the scope of protections can help create a work environment that supports the needs of pregnant workers and new mothers.

Addressing poverty and wealth inequality is fundamental to promoting reproductive justice for African American women. Poverty significantly impacts health outcomes throughout an individual's lifespan, and it is crucial to address this issue through economic policies. Increasing the minimum wage can lift families from poverty and provide financial stability for pregnant workers and new mothers. Ensuring equal pay for equal work helps bridge the wage gap that disproportionately affects women, particularly women of color. More progressive tax policies can help redistribute wealth and create a more equitable society.

Supporting pregnant workers and new mothers requires a multifaceted approach that includes policies such as paid leave, affordable childcare, enforcement of anti-discrimination laws, and economic measures to address poverty and wealth inequality. These initiatives can create a supportive environment for African American women and contribute to better health outcomes for both mothers and infants.

2. Adopt a comprehensive paid family and medical leave

Regrettably, the availability of paid leave for workers in the United States is limited, leaving many individuals needing more support to care for themselves or their loved ones, including newborn infants. A mere 17 percent of American workers have access to paid leave, highlighting the widespread lack of this crucial benefit. Consequently, a significant majority of mothers employed during pregnancy are compelled to return to work within a mere six months after giving birth. Shockingly, nearly 1 in 4 mothers are forced to resume work in less than two weeks after delivering their infants.

The statistics demonstrate the insufficiency of paid leave policies in the United States, resulting in inadequate time for mothers to recover from childbirth and adequately bond with their newborns.

The absence of sufficient paid leave forces new mothers to face immense pressure to return to work prematurely, potentially jeopardizing their health and the well-being of their infants. The lack of supportive policies contributes to working mothers' challenges, particularly those in vulnerable socioeconomic situations, including African American women disproportionately affected by poverty and limited access to resources.

Expanding and strengthening paid leave policies becomes an urgent necessity to address these concerning realities. By enacting comprehensive and inclusive paid family and medical leave legislation, more workers would have the opportunity to take the time they need to care for their health and that of their loved ones, including newborn infants. Adequate paid leave would alleviate financial burdens, offer job security, and enable mothers to prioritize their physical and emotional well-being during the critical postpartum period.

Furthermore, extending the duration of paid leave and ensuring its accessibility to a broader range of workers would significantly improve outcomes for working mothers and their infants. Recognizing the unique needs and challenges African American women face, targeted efforts should be made to address the specific barriers they encounter, such as socioeconomic disparities and racial biases.

Ultimately, expanding and enhancing paid leave policies are crucial steps toward establishing a more equitable and supportive environment for working mothers, enabling them to prioritize their health, bond with their infants, and contribute positively to the workforce.

By prioritizing the well-being of mothers and infants through comprehensive paid leave policies, society can take significant strides in addressing health disparities and promoting the overall welfare of families.

3. Support breastfeeding

New mothers employed in low-wage jobs, manual labor, or the service industry, which disproportionately includes women of color, often face additional challenges in accessing breastfeeding support.

Despite existing policies supporting breastfeeding mothers, disparities persist in breastfeeding rates. Policymakers must take further action to incentivize the implementation of these existing policies and ensure adequate time and space for new mothers to express breast milk while at work.

Under the Affordable Care Act (ACA), workplace support for breastfeeding was mandated, including employers providing break time and private space for mothers to express breast milk. These provisions enable mothers to continue breastfeeding after returning to work. Additionally, the ACA requires insurance coverage for breastfeeding support, counseling, and supplies without cost-sharing, which is vital for reducing disparities in breastfeeding rates, particularly along racial and economic lines. Women covered by Medicaid and those participating in the Women, Infants, and Children (WIC) program also have access to breastfeeding support and education.

However, despite these critical provisions, more must be done to ensure equitable access to breastfeeding support for all workers, regardless of employer size or industry. Policymakers can play a pivotal role by expanding the scope of these requirements to encompass all workers.

By extending the coverage of workplace breastfeeding supports beyond the current limitations, policymakers can bridge the gaps in access faced by women in low-wage and service industry jobs, where support is often lacking.

Efforts to promote breastfeeding among working mothers must be intersectional, taking into account the specific challenges women of color face in these industries. Targeted initiatives and culturally sensitive support can help address disparities and ensure all breastfeeding mothers have the resources and accommodations they need to succeed.

In summary, while policies such as those mandated by the ACA have laid the groundwork for workplace breastfeeding support, disparities exist, particularly for women in low-wage jobs and industries that predominantly employ women of color.

Policymakers should expand and strengthen these policies to ensure comprehensive support for all workers, regardless of employer size or industry. By doing so, society can promote equity in breastfeeding rates and improve mothers' and infants' overall health and well-being.

Ensure humane treatment of pregnant and postpartum women in the criminal justice system.

Women of color face a disproportionate representation within the criminal justice system. This means that a higher percentage of women from these communities become involved in the legal system than their model in the overall population. Disturbingly, nearly 80 percent of incarcerated women are mothers, with most being single mothers. Many of these women are imprisoned for minor offenses. Additionally, incarcerated women of color often come from low-income backgrounds, have experienced violence, and are predisposed to trauma.

The impact of incarceration on pregnant women is particularly concerning. Incarcerated pregnant women face risks to their physical and mental health and heightened vulnerability to violence and substance abuse. This creates a distressing environment that can negatively affect the mother and her unborn child.

The overrepresentation of women of color in the criminal justice system has far-reaching consequences, extending beyond the individuals themselves to their children. Parental incarceration is classified as an Adverse Childhood Experience (ACE), which refers to traumatic events during childhood that can have long-lasting effects on health and well-being.

Sadly, due to decades of racial discrimination and discriminatory sentencing practices within the criminal justice system, African American children are more than twice as likely as non-Hispanic white children to have an incarcerated parent or guardian.

The impact of parental incarceration on children is profound and multifaceted. It can disrupt family stability, financial security, and access to resources.

Children may experience emotional distress, educational challenges, and an increased likelihood of involvement in the criminal justice system themselves. The cycle of incarceration becomes perpetuated, exacerbating existing racial disparities and contributing to intergenerational inequities.

To address these issues, it is crucial to implement comprehensive reforms within the criminal justice system. This includes reevaluating sentencing practices, promoting alternatives to incarceration for nonviolent offenses, and investing in rehabilitative programs that address the underlying factors contributing to criminal behavior.

Additionally, providing support and resources to incarcerated mothers, such as access to parenting programs, mental health services, and assistance with reentry into the community, can help mitigate the harmful effects of incarceration on both mothers and their children.

Moreover, efforts must be made to tackle the root causes of the overrepresentation of women of color in the criminal justice system. This involves addressing systemic racism, socioeconomic disparities, and the lack of access to opportunities and resources in marginalized communities.

By implementing comprehensive criminal justice reforms and addressing the underlying social and economic factors contributing to racial disparities, society can create a more equitable system that supports the well-being of women of color, their children, and their communities.

Implement Tax Supports For Families

Tax credits play a crucial role in supporting families during a child's birth. However, the current Child Tax Credit system falls short, as it is not accessible to families with insufficient earnings. This exclusion disproportionately affects the country's lowest-income families, many headed by women of color. To truly invest in these families, it is necessary to enhance and improve the Child Tax Credit in several ways.

Firstly, making the Child Tax Credit fully refundable is essential. Currently, families with low or no taxable income may not receive the full benefit of the credit. By making it fully refundable, all eligible families, regardless of their income level, could access the credit in its entirety, providing them with much-needed financial support during the critical period after the birth of a child.

Additionally, modifying the Child Tax Credit distribution method can have a significant impact. Rather than receiving the credit as a lump sum during tax filing season, providing the option to receive it every month would be beneficial. This approach would enable families to promptly cover essential expenses such as formula and diapers, alleviating the financial strain associated with caring for an infant.

Furthermore, recognizing the unique needs of families with young children and providing an additional boost for families with children under the age of six is crucial. This age group requires specific resources and support, and tailoring the Child Tax Credit to provide increased assistance during these early years can significantly benefit families, especially those facing economic challenges.

Expanding and improving the Child Tax Credit in these ways would positively impact families, particularly those headed by women of color who often face more significant financial barriers.

It would help address disparities and provide much-needed financial relief during the critical period following the birth of a child. By investing in these families through an enhanced Child Tax Credit, society can promote more excellent economic stability and support the well-being of children and their caregivers.

Eliminate Harmful Work Requirements

Traditional Medicaid and Medicaid expansion should be implemented without the inclusion of work requirements, as these policies disproportionately harm women of color. Work requirements serve as harsh time limits that offer no real investment in job creation or wage increases.

They may even hinder individuals' ability to find employment. The National Academy of Sciences has found that such policies are "at least as likely to increase as to decrease poverty," indicating their limited effectiveness.

Despite having the highest labor force participation rates among women, African American women face higher rates of unemployment and more extended periods of joblessness than their white counterparts.

They are also likelier to work in low-wage jobs, often with unstable schedules and irregular hours. These jobs are particularly vulnerable to coverage losses when work requirements are in place. As a result, women of color may risk losing access to vital healthcare services.

For instance, in Arkansas, a state that recently implemented a work requirement of 80 hours per month, over 18,000 individuals have already lost their Medicaid coverage due to these requirements. Alarmingly, fewer than 2,000 of those individuals have been able to reenroll, potentially leaving them without essential healthcare.

It is essential to recognize that work requirements must address the underlying challenges individuals seeking healthcare assistance face. Instead of providing meaningful support, these policies create additional barriers for those already facing economic hardships and limited job opportunities.

To ensure equitable access to healthcare, removing work requirements from Medicaid programs is crucial. Focusing on job creation, wage improvements, and economic policies that address systemic barriers would be more effective in supporting individuals, including women of color, in their pursuit of stable employment and access to vital healthcare services.

Expanding Medicaid coverage without work requirements would ensure that individuals receive the necessary healthcare support without jeopardizing their access due to arbitrary employment criteria.

This approach aligns with principles of equity and recognizes the systemic barriers faced by women of color in the labor market. By implementing inclusive healthcare policies, society can take significant steps towards improving the well-being of all individuals, particularly those who have historically faced disproportionate barriers to healthcare access.

Throughout this extensive exploration, we have delved deep into the complex realities of being pregnant and black in America. The journey of black mothers-to-be is marred by adversity, strength, and a relentless pursuit of justice. From conception to birthing, these women face many challenges rooted in historical injustices, systemic prejudices, and deeply ingrained biases.

As we conclude this journey, it is paramount to reflect on the urgent call for change, to scrutinize the systemic issues perpetuating these disparities, and to envision a future where every expectant mother, regardless of race, can embrace the joys of pregnancy with dignity, unwavering support, and equitable access to quality care.

1. Unveiling the Disparities: A System Stacked Against Black Mothers

Our exploration has brought to light the stark disparities experienced by black pregnant women in America. Extensive research has consistently revealed the uncomfortable truth of racial inequality in maternal healthcare. Black women suffer from higher pregnancy-related complications, maternal mortality, and infant mortality rates than their white counterparts. These disparities are the product of numerous factors, including limited access to healthcare, implicit biases within the healthcare system, socioeconomic inequalities, and environmental influences. Acknowledging and confronting these disparities is the critical first step toward effecting meaningful change.

2. Systemic Biases and the Healthcare System: Demanding Equitable Care

Implicit biases embedded within the healthcare system contribute significantly to the unequal treatment and care received by black pregnant women. Unconscious stereotypes and prejudices healthcare providers hold can lead to dismissive attitudes, delayed diagnoses, and substandard care.

Cultivating cultural competence among healthcare professionals, promoting diversity within the medical workforce, and implementing policies that actively dismantle bias and discrimination is essential.

By fostering an inclusive and compassionate environment, we can ensure that every pregnant mother receives the care and support she deserves, regardless of race or ethnicity.

3. The Role of Prenatal Care and Education: Empowering Mothers-to-Be

Accessible and quality prenatal care is vital in promoting positive maternal and infant health outcomes. Unfortunately, pregnant black women often encounter significant barriers to adequate prenatal care. These barriers include limited financial resources, lack of transportation, and a scarcity of healthcare providers in their communities.

Addressing these systemic barriers necessitates a multifaceted approach, including expanding access to affordable healthcare, increasing the number of healthcare providers in underserved areas, and implementing community-based programs that offer education and support to expectant mothers. Empowering black mothers-to-be with knowledge and resources can lead to healthier pregnancies and improved birth outcomes.

4. Advocacy and Policy Reform: Amplifying the Voices of Change

Creating lasting change requires amplifying the voices of those directly affected and engaging in advocacy efforts that confront the systemic issues black pregnant women face. Grassroots organizations, community leaders, and policy advocates are pivotal in raising awareness, mobilizing communities, and advocating for policy reform.

Comprehensive reforms are needed at all levels, from local communities to federal institutions, to ensure equitable access to healthcare, reduce racial disparities, and dismantle the systemic barriers that impede the well-being of black pregnant women. Supporting legislative initiatives, increasing funding for research and programs, and holding institutions accountable are crucial steps toward building a more just and inclusive healthcare system.

5. Shifting Cultural Narratives: Celebrating Black Motherhood

Transforming the narrative surrounding black motherhood is a decisive step toward addressing black pregnant women's challenges in America. Media representation, education, and public discourse are pivotal in shaping perceptions and dismantling harmful stereotypes. By highlighting diverse stories and experiences, promoting positive models of black motherhood, and challenging prevailing narratives, we can reshape societal perceptions and foster a culture that values and supports black mothers-to-be.

In conclusion, our exploration of being pregnant and black in America has illuminated the profound challenges black mothers-to-be face while highlighting the urgent need for comprehensive change. We must carry black pregnant women's stories, experiences, and struggles as a reminder of the pressing need for transformation.

May their voices ignite a collective determination to create a future where every expectant mother can embark on the pregnancy journey with hope, dignity, and unwavering support. Together, we can reshape the narrative, address the disparities, and build a society that cherishes and safeguards the well-being of all its mothers.

The path may be long, but by working collaboratively, embracing empathy, and advocating for change, we can foster a future that upholds every expectant mother's rights and dignity, regardless of race or ethnicity.

Know This!

There's Segregation and Intimidation Even Among The Blacks.

Discrimination, unfortunately, knows no bounds and can manifest itself within various communities, including among people who share the same skin color. While it may be disheartening, it is not entirely surprising that discrimination based on class and social standing exists even within the Black community. This form of discrimination highlights the intricate complexities and power dynamics that can arise when wealth and fame come into play.

In this context, the discrimination centers around economic disparities and the influence that money and fame wield within society. Those who possess substantial wealth and enjoy widespread recognition often find themselves in positions of privilege, which can lead to the abuse of power and the mistreatment of others.

Within the Black community, the impact of class discrimination can be particularly painful. It underscores the unfortunate reality that financial success does not always translate into a dismantling of systemic inequalities. Instead, it can sometimes result in the perpetuation of social hierarchies and the creation of exclusive circles, where individuals vie for superiority based on their wealth, fame, or connections.

The concept of having the "whole system in their pockets" further emphasizes the deep-rooted influence that individuals with significant resources can yield. They may exploit their connections and financial leverage to shape institutions, sway public opinion, or gain preferential treatment. This abuse of power can marginalize those who are not as financially fortunate, creating divisions and exacerbating the disparities that already exist within the Black community.

Personal experiences of such discrimination can be profoundly impactful and can vary widely. Some may face exclusion from social circles or professional opportunities due to their perceived lack of financial status. Others may encounter subtle forms of mistreatment or condescension, where their achievements are diminished or disregarded in comparison to those with greater wealth or fame.

It is crucial to recognize and address these issues within the Black community, just as it is important to combat discrimination in any form.

By fostering dialogue, promoting inclusivity, and working towards a more equitable society, we can strive to break down these barriers and create a world where all individuals are valued based on their character and abilities rather than their socioeconomic status.

Read on as I share my own personal experience with discrimination among people of the same race and color:

When I found out I was pregnant with my first baby in Nigeria, I quickly realized that giving birth here was primarily about class rather than race. The distinction between the rich and the poor became starkly apparent when it came to choosing a healthcare facility.

Wealthy individuals often opted for private hospitals, where doctors owned their practices and the entire operation was significantly more expensive compared to the government-owned general hospitals.

Initially, I decided to seek prenatal care at a private hospital close to where I lived. It was convenient, just a 5-minute drive or a 15-minute walk away. The doctor there had over 30 years of experience and seemed skilled at what he did. However, after going there for the first six months of my pregnancy, I decided to switch to the government hospital.

One of the reasons behind my decision was the fact that private hospitals were believed to prefer performing cesarean sections (C-sections) during childbirth because they could charge significantly more for the procedure, around $1500 compared to just $200 at the general hospital. In contrast, at the government hospital, the doctors had no personal gain in recommending unnecessary C-sections. They had more than one doctor on call at all times, working together to ensure the well-being of the patients.

What I loved most about the general hospital was the support and community I found there. They held regular meetings and teachings for pregnant women, typically two or three times a week. During these sessions, we would sing, dance, and share our concerns, providing advice on what to do when feeling a certain way or what to eat. The nurses would distribute mosquito nets, as they were particularly concerned about pregnant women contracting malaria. They preferred prevention over medication and only allowed the use of multivitamins and folic acids during pregnancy. They would only prescribe medication if you were truly sick, and even then, it would typically be limited to approved treatments for pregnant women, which became available only around the seventh month of pregnancy.

Overall, my experience highlighted the disparities in healthcare access and practices based on class in Nigeria. While private hospitals offered convenience and experienced doctors, they were often associated with a higher likelihood of unnecessary C-sections due to financial incentives.

On the other hand, general hospitals provided a sense of community and a focus on holistic care, prioritizing prevention and offering more affordable treatment options. It was eye-opening to witness the contrast and made me appreciate the benefits of a healthcare system that considers the well-being of all individuals, regardless of their socioeconomic status.

I absolutely adored the singing sessions during the prenatal meetings at the general hospital. It was such a joy to meet diverse individuals from various walks of life and make friends along the way. Connecting with other pregnant women who were going through similar experiences provided a sense of relief and camaraderie.

When my water broke and I rushed to the hospital, I initially spent around three hours in the labor room, but my contractions weren't strong enough for me to be admitted. However, in the early hours of the following day, my water broke again, and I returned to the labor room.

Ultimately, I ended up having a C-section because my cervix didn't dilate as expected, and I was getting tired. The doctor who attended to me remained incredibly optimistic and encouraging throughout the process. He assured me that I could handle it, considering my height and age were favorable factors.

He waited until the very last moment before we made the decision to proceed with the C-section. Unfortunately, I missed one of the regular meetings during this time, but I found solace and support in joining a group on the Peanut app, where pregnant women like me connected for encouragement and shared their feelings.

At Grady Hospital, there was a group of doctors from Emory University who took care of me. One particular doctor always made me feel special. Whenever she entered the room, she would compliment my dress and appearance.

She once mentioned that even if she hadn't read my case file or knew who she was coming to meet, she would recognize me because I always looked good for my appointments. I made a conscious effort throughout my pregnancy not to let the challenges weigh me down.

Regardless of any news or results I received, I held onto hope. During one of my visits, a receptionist called me aside as I was leaving the hospital and praised my dress, saying I looked incredibly beautiful with my pregnancy, even though I was already 38 weeks along.

Throughout my pregnancy journey, I maintained a positive mindset and believed that everything would turn out okay. I made sure to show up and present myself confidently, regardless of any uncertainties. I am immensely grateful that my optimism paid off and that I had a supportive and friendly environment to navigate through this transformative experience.

As you now know, discrimination, segregation, scrutiny, stereotyping, Intimidation and other ills of the society are to be treated from within. Within ourselves. Ask yourself if you are ready for that change — a change that would influence another person to change

Personal Notes

I want to believe with every fiber of my being that my story and research will reach the hearts and minds of those who possess the power to implement the long-awaited dream of every black pregnant woman around the world.

This plea is not only directed to the expectant mothers out there but to all who can understand the profound significance of this message. I yearn for you to perceive it for what it truly is—a peaceful but resolute protest that seeks to protect and nurture the lives of our unborn children, and to finally grant us the boundless joy that comes with being a mother.

To all the mothers out there, I want this heartfelt plea to reach you as well. Together, let us stand unwavering in our strength and resilience, for we bear the weight of hope upon our shoulders. We envision a future where our children are born into this world with ease, unburdened by the inequalities that have plagued us for far too long.

We dream of a world where our freedom to live and thrive is not just a fleeting promise, but an undeniable truth protected by the hands of justice and righteousness.

Allow me to introduce myself once more, for names carry stories, and stories hold power. My name is Temitope Oluyemo, a dedicated real estate agent hailing from the state of Georgia. I am also a triumphant entrepreneur, having navigated the turbulent seas of life with determination and grace.

But above all, I am a mother—blessed with the privilege of raising three extraordinary boys who have captured my heart and soul. It is through them that I have discovered the true essence of motherhood—the boundless love, the unwavering devotion, and the relentless pursuit of providing them with the best life possible.

Dear fellow mothers, let us forge a path of unity and solidarity, where our collective voices become an unstoppable force for change. May our longing for a better world be the catalyst that ignites the flame of transformation within society. Let us not falter or waver, for our dreams of a brighter tomorrow for our children deserve nothing less than our unwavering commitment.

As we raise our voices, may they resonate with compassion, understanding, and empathy, reaching out to those whose hearts have remained closed to our struggles. For it is through love and understanding that we can bridge the gaps that divide us, creating a society where the color of our skin holds no bearing on the opportunities and care we receive.

Together, let us envision a future where the journey of motherhood transcends the barriers of race, where black pregnant women are cherished and supported without question. Let us strive for a world where the arrival of a new life is celebrated universally, unburdened by the shadows of discrimination and bias.

To every mother who reads these words, may you find solace in the knowledge that you are not alone. Our shared experiences, triumphs, and challenges bind us together in an unbreakable bond. Let us continue to draw strength from one another as we march forward, unwavering in our pursuit of a world that treasures the sacredness of motherhood.

And so, I implore you, my fellow warriors of love, stand tall, for our cause is just. Let our voices echo through the corridors of power, touching the hearts of those who possess the ability to effect change.

For the longing wish of every black pregnant woman, every mother, and every unborn child is intertwined within our collective plea—a plea for a future where every child is born into a world that embraces them with open arms, and where the joy of motherhood knows no bounds.

With boundless hope and unwavering determination,

-Temitope Oluyemo.